A GOOD NIGHT'S SLEEP

Anna Wahlgren

A GOOD NIGHT'S SLEEP

English translation by
Bruce Junkin

FÖRLAG ANNA WAHLGREN AB

The opinions and advice in this book are just that – my opinions and advice. Some of these may be contrary to professional or government-endorsed advice that you receive on child rearing and parenting and so it is up to you – the parent, the carer, the reader, to decide how to use all of this information. In other words, any reliance upon any information in this book shall be taken at your own risk. The author and publisher cannot be held liable for any claims, actions or demands resulting from any person undertaking any or all of the recommendations, information, suggestions or advice in this book.

Anna Wahlgren
Author and International Publisher

(Förlag Anna Wahlgren AB)

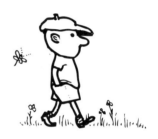

Swedish original title: Internationella sova hela natten
English translation: Bruce Junkin
Editing: Anna Wahlgren, Lisa Waldron
Cover: Christian von Essen
Author photo: Lieselotte van der Meijs
Publishing company: Förlag Anna Wahlgren AB
Typesetting and layout: Manne Svensson
Print: Swepo Grafiska
ISBN: 978-91-977736-1-4

TABLE OF CONTENTS:

I.

A GOOD NIGHT'S SLEEP
A FEW INTRODUCTORY WORDS

Dear Mom, dear Dad,

Are you up all night? Are you so tired that you fear for your sanity? Does it seem as though the whole family is about to crash and burn?

Perhaps you can recognize yourself in the following lines from an anxious father:

We have an adorable little girl of four months. The problem is her sleep pattern and getting her to sleep the whole night.

She only falls asleep after a lengthy ordeal that involves breastfeeding, rocking and much fussing.

Unfortunately, she wakes up crying time after time during the night, and my wife has to bear most of the burden, since I work long hours.

Even the days are a problem. She sleeps a maximum of 20–30 minutes at a stretch, three times a day at the most.

I am very worried about her mother's health. I can see that this is wearing her down and she is not feeling well.

I try to help out as much as I can, but I am reaching the end of my tether.

You are our last hope.

Don't despair! The help you seek is in the book you are holding in your hand. The *Good-Night's-Sleep Cure* will enable you to help your child sleep soundly, peacefully and continuously, not for five, six or seven hours, but for twelve. Or eleven, eleven and a half if that suits you better.

You will break out of the vicious cycle you find yourself in, a cycle where lack of sleep affects every aspect of your life – your appetite, your ability to work, your *joie de vivre*, your love – and in only a few days your lives will be back on track.

The good nights will mean good days. Your little baby will be stronger and happier. Your own powers, your self-esteem and your self-confidence will grow as your baby's lust for life blossoms.

The set routines will make your existence simple. The *Good-Night's-Sleep Cure* will give you and your whole family a freedom of movement that you are probably too tired to even dream about now.

From a now well-rested mother:
If you haven't been there yourself, you cannot understand how exhausting never being allowed to sleep properly is. By the same token, no one understands what a godsend Anna's cure is for so many parents of small children like us.

One day I went grocery shopping, bought what I needed, paid at the cash, and then left all my purchases at the store and arrived back home empty-handed. Once I got into the house, I couldn't figure out where all the food had gone. There is a limit to how tired you can get.

I don't understand how I/we managed before you came along. We can't thank you enough, dear Anna!

My husband didn't believe in the Good-Night's-Sleep Cure *when we began, but oh is he a convert now!*

Not being able to sleep is agony. Sleep deprivation is a tried and tested method of torture. If human beings are deprived of sleep for long enough, they will be prepared to go along with just about anything. You don't need to go along with anything any longer. Nor does your little baby.

The whole family must be allowed to sleep if life is to be as good as it should be when you have a little baby to enjoy. For little babies should be enjoyed – and enjoy themselves!

In just four nights, three days and a follow-up week, the *Good-Night's-Sleep Cure* will give you your life back.

The mother of little Philip, seven months, wrote to me:

I love our new life and I am so incredibly grateful for it. I went from being an exhausted mother who didn't really have the strength to do anything to being an alert and happy Mom, who has more than enough energy to socialize with her son, her husband and her friends. And I can spend some time on myself because I really have the time now!

My husband and I are so proud of our son. When we go to bed, we still marvel over how easy everything is. Can it really be true?

I tend to take the bull by the horns, while my husband is a little less sure of himself. Philip figured that out immediately. So I was the one who took charge of the cure nights and the follow-up week. I was then able to get my husband enthused, since he saw that this really worked. Now it doesn't matter who puts Philip to bed – me, my husband or grandma – any of us can do it.

I also want to raise a toast to the goodnight laugh! It is so important. It gets Philip to associate going to bed with something fun. He actually gets CHEERFUL when we go into his bedroom. And we do too. The going-to-bed procedure becomes a great way to round off the day.

Once we have put Philip to bed in the evening, I find I can't wait for him to wake up again because he has become such a sweet, cheery, energetic little guy who just radiates positive energy. Of course he was wonderful even before the cure, but I was so tired back then and Philip could be whiny, since neither of us was sleeping very well.

He has become quite a little glutton too!

To those of you who are worried about dispensing with the pacifier (I know I was), don't be! Infants forget all about it after the first night. There was a time when Philip always had a pacifier in his mouth, but now he doesn't want it. I brought out the pacifier again just to see what he would do. I put it in his mouth, but he spat it out and started to play with it instead!

I hope these words give people a bit of a lift and some inspiration. If we can do it, everyone can!

And being allowed to sleep is so divine.

Dear Mom, dear Dad,

Once you decide to run with the *Good-Night's-Sleep Cure*, good times are coming. Tens of thousands of parents of small children can attest to this.

I know you don't dare believe this yet. You don't believe that it will work on *your* baby.

But listen to little Maria's mom:
Today, June 4, 2006, I am sitting down to write something I never believed that I would have the privilege of writing.

We have a daughter, Maria, who is just over 15 months old. Since last Easter, we have been following the Good-Night's-Sleep Cure *to the letter, and the results have surpassed our wildest expectations.*

Anna Wahlgren wrote to us that good times were coming, but we didn't realize how good!

Before the cure, Maria would wake up 10 to 14 times a night. My husband and I worked in shifts, half conscious and bleary-eyed. We prepared at least three bottles of formula per night and we must have had ten pacifiers in her bed, so we could lay our hands on one as soon as she woke up. We were both at breaking point, since we were never allowed to sleep. We were close to divorcing.

But then we were given a tip about this fantastic cure! Words cannot describe how our lives have changed since we began this cure. Now Maria sleeps 11 hours a night plus two naps during the day.

In spite of her getting masses of new teeth during this period, as well as having a cold and a fever, the cure has worked. She seldom if ever wakes up during the night. If she does wake up, she falls back to sleep on her own. We occasionally have to recite a good night rhyme, but we don't even get out of bed.

For a few weeks, we had to suffer through the pre-dawn hours, but I soon decided that I wasn't going to put up with her waking up around 5.00 or 5.30 a.m. So I began to set my alarm for a time just before I knew she would wake up so that I could be outside her door the instant she came to and recite a so-called reassurance rhyme. She never had the chance to cry herself into a frenzy. It worked. Now she wakes up at around 6.30, which is when her dad has to get up for work.

When Maria goes down for a nap during the day, all we have to do is put her in the carriage and place a thin blanket over the hood. She is asleep in five minutes. We never have to push the carriage around or push it back and forth. She gets the message.

When we get together with other parents with young children, they often cast jealous glances at us and tell us how lucky we are to have such a fantastic baby who falls asleep so easily. When we try to tell them that this is perfectly feasible for their kids too, they don't really seem to listen. Why I can't understand?! They immediately come back with a bunch of counter-arguments. Babies should not sleep by themselves, they want to read bedtime stories to their babies, and on and on it goes. But we read stories and look at pictures with our child too, but in another room and before it is time for bed. None of this seems to register.

One other thing that I don't understand. Why isn't this fantastic cure recommended by children's clinics? All we were told was that the Controlled Crying Method was our only option. They even wanted to send us to a child psychologist because our daughter never slept. It is just so SICK!

As Anna also writes, this method gives permanent results. We notice this when we use our fabulous baby sitter, who is well acquainted with our routines. All she has to do is check the note on the fridge, and she knows exactly what to do.

Before this cure, I thought I would never have another child. But now that I know how to get infants sleep all night and my bedroom is kid-free, who knows?

I hope these lines will give parents who are thinking of trying this cure the heads-up. IT WORKS!

NB. All the questions and comments from parents in this book are authentic, unsolicited quotes, however some names have been changed to protect and respect the privacy of the children concerned. The quotes can be found at www.annawahlgren.com in the section "Life after the Cure – An Encouragement" ("Livet efter kuren – en uppmuntran"). Please note, however, that at the time of printing, this section of the website is only available in Swedish.

WHY DOES THE GOOD-NIGHT'S-SLEEP CURE WORK?

The *Good-Night's-Sleep Cure* is just that – a cure – a remedy for young children who need help to be able to sleep soundly and continuously all through the night.

The cure works on all children with sleep problems because young children, just like all beings of flesh and blood, need and want to sleep at night.

We all want to sleep peacefully. Children are no exception.

The *Good-Night's-Sleep Cure* can be administered to all little people who don't see eye-to-eye with the Sandman from four months on.

There is no upper age limit.

The father of eight-month-old Allen had this to say about the cure:
Until he was four months old, Allen slept unusually well at night and we were beginning to think that things were going to stay that way. Of course, that was when the problems started. To cut a long story short, we didn't sleep a whole night for more than four months. He would wake up five to ten times a night. We would feed him, rock him, bring him to our bed, put him back in his own...

We were feeling the strain to say the least. This affected not only us, but also our five-year-old daughter and of course our work.

We contacted our local children's clinic, where we spoke to a nurse who was very understanding, but she couldn't help us. We called pediatrics at our local hospital, but they had no advice to give us either. We spoke to a child psychologist, who I'm sure suspected we were not caring for our son properly. No one could help us.

Quite by chance, I wandered onto Anna's homepage when I was surfing and looking for parents who had problems similar to ours. I immediately got the feeling that this was some kind of turning point. I read about the cure and the wolf analogy, and I thought, Good Lord, here is someone who has actually pondered over WHY children wake up at night, not just how you get them to go to sleep.

We bought A Good Night's Sleep *a couple of days later, and the more we read, the more convinced we were that this was the common sense advice that we had sought but failed to find from the so-called experts. The only controversial point – that children as a rule sleep better on their stomachs – we had already figured out. From the time he was able to turn over by himself, Allen has always slept on his stomach and we never tried to change this.*

Almost two weeks ago, we started the cure. The first night was hard going. But from the second night on, we noticed a huge difference, and on the fourth night, Allen slept continuously from eight in the evening to five in the morning. Talk about chalk and cheese! We thought that if we could keep this up, we were home free. If we could sleep until 5.00 a.m., that would be bearable and we could adapt.

But as we continued the cure, things got better and better. Just last night, Allen slept from 7.30 in the evening to 7.00 in the morning without waking up once, which was exactly the schedule that we had set up.

We are well rested, we have more energy, and we get more out of life. And suddenly Allen has begun to eat like a horse, whereas before he would just spit out his food. The transformation has been fantastic. It's hard to grasp that just three weeks ago, we weren't getting more than a couple of hours' uninterrupted sleep a night.

There is absolutely no fault we can find with this cure. It has worked perfectly for us, and I can only encourage those who are in the same bind that we once were to give it a shot. The results are simply unbeatable.

Our warmest thanks to Anna, who without even knowing us has taught us so much!

The *Good-Night's-Sleep Cure* has been developed in close cooperation with the hundreds upon hundreds of infants with sleep problems that I personally, over the last thirty years, have been able to help get a good night's sleep.

The underlying principle of the *Good-Night's-Sleep Cure* is simple and well grounded: *calm the children where they are lying.*

And this must be done safely, proactively and preventively.

A mother writes:

Thanks Anna for being there and having the courage to speak up! The Controlled Crying method was far too cruel for us.

The Good-Night's-Sleep Cure *was the turning point for our one-year-old. We didn't 'experiment'. We took charge and laid down the law. At night everyone sleeps like logs!*

We had done our homework of course. You shouldn't have to think too hard in the middle of the night.

Result? Twelve hours' sleep a night after one week. That was two and a half years ago and no changes yet.

The *Good-Night's-Sleep Cure* is the solution for those of you who, with the best of intentions, have caused your young child's sleep problems.

You are buckling under the strain of sleep deprivation. Because you are in the throes of exhaustion and desperation yourself, perhaps you can understand how your child feels.

You want to put an end to an unsustainable situation. And it won't be difficult. The *Good-Night's-Sleep Cure* can be seen through by anyone, you included, no matter how tired and despondent you have been feeling for God knows how many months.

Just making the decision will enable you to draw on reserves you didn't know you had. Decisions lead to action and fixity of purpose. Nothing dispels feelings of powerlessness like decisive action.

A mother tells me:

My social life was zero from the time our son was born until last week. My mother and my in-laws were the only people I had the strength to see – sometimes.

During a 'good' night we might have squared five or six hours sleep, and if we were really lucky, two of them were continuous. (Very rare.)

No one – and I mean NO ONE – understood how tough we had it, since no one we know had gone through what we had to contend with. Those people who said they had 'difficult' kids claimed that it was normal that young children slept badly. Their kids woke up all of THREE(!!!) times per night. God, heaven on earth compared to what we were going through, I thought to myself!

I know I shouldn't wallow in self-pity, but with everyone telling me that my situation was normal, I felt like the world's biggest loser because I couldn't do the super Mom thing. All I had the strength to do was stay home and feed my child, dress my child and put my child to bed – the bare necessities in other words. (As for playing with my child, that just wasn't part of my universe.) I was so tired I was in tears most of the time. My husband and I would fight over the most trivial things. I didn't have the strength to tend to any of my own needs. I couldn't understand why this was, since everyone else with children seemed to manage just fine!

After countless appeals to my local children's clinic, I was finally given referrals to a child psychologist and a doctor. There was a four-week wait to see the psychologist. The doctor gave me a prescription for tranquilizers – FOR THE CHILD!

We were both suffering from major burn-out. I took the first few nights and my husband took the days. It took about five nights before we got any indication that this cure actually worked. So we spent five days and nights in limbo caught between hope and doubt. During the follow-up week, we actually slept through the night without having to intervene at all. I WEPT TEARS OF PURE JOY!

Now, after a week of blissful sleep, words cannot express how happy I am. I still wake up two or three times a night when my little guy comes to and peeps a little, but he goes back to sleep BY HIMSELF in a minute or so!

So I send my best wishes and a little of my new-found strength to all of you who are thinking of embarking on this cure. I know you can do it because if our little one can get his sleeping act together, yours can too! GUARANTEED!

It's just a matter of believing in what you are doing. Your child will be able to sleep. And that is what you all want.

Words of encouragement from a mother:
I've got to get this on the record! I challenge all you doubting Thomases out there to apply the Good-Night's-Sleep Cure*!*

We had problems with our 14-month-old daughter's constant wakefulness. It put a strain on our patience and our strength, and in the end we were just too weary to deal with the problem. We thought that she was just going through a 'phase' and that it would soon pass. But this 'phase' became permanent. Some nights were better than others of course, and she would only wake up two or three times. But then the situation would deteriorate and it was back to square one. Our daughter woke up constantly, sometimes staying awake for hours at a time. Nothing helped!

We were advised to let her sleep with us, which we did. No effect at all! I stopped breastfeeding altogether to see if it would help, but that didn't work either. We also tried the Controlled Crying Method, but that was unbearable – she would scream until she retched, and eventually fell into exhausted unconsciousness, only to wake up again... and again and again.

Finally we said ENOUGH! I had heard of the 'Anna Wahlgren Method', but when I started to read about it, I realized that I hadn't really understood what it was all about. We read up on our subject and made our decision. And it felt so right!

So we rolled up our sleeves and got to work. Of course, there were a few trying nights and the odd setback (as Anna warned us there would be), but we tried to make the best of things – a mattress on the floor outside the door and some reading material. And it worked! Our daughter now sleeps all night, and I sometimes think I have died and gone to heaven! We have a lot of sleep to catch up on! Of course she sometimes wakes up before she is supposed to, but she lies in her bed and babbles for a while, and then drops off again all by herself.

Thank you Anna with all my heart – you have saved our whole family! Now we can really enjoy parenthood and life again. We are no longer burdened with the prospect of yet another sleepless night. Never being allowed to sleep is such torment.

Our daughter is on top of the world and really enjoys being put to bed.

Nature's imperative dictates that children shall develop and grow and continue to do so no matter how exhausted they are. Their lust for life is what drives them. Their will to live is unstoppable.

But if they are denied sleep, they don't have the strength to enjoy their inexorable lust for life for very long. They become whiny, clingy and anxious. But they can still smile with a bit of coaxing. That lust for life, courageous and unwavering, shines through in their smiles.

It is easy for an adult to draw the erroneous conclusion that everything is as it should be as long as the infant seems basically happy. It is easy to ignore the pallor, the dark circles under the eyes, the clingy whininess and the corrosive anxiety as long as the child continues to gain weight and can be coaxed into a smile.

That mental prerequisite – a lust for life – is hardwired into every child. This fact does not, however, give us a *carte blanche* to ignore young children's tremendous need for sleep.

A new mother tells her story:

When our child was seven weeks old, night feedings had escalated to four or five. That was four or five half-hour sessions – every night. The day began officially at six, when he wanted breakfast. Both of us were half dead from fatigue. He cried and rubbed his eyes after his meal, but he couldn't go back to sleep. It was the same story at six at night. Whimpering, dreary evenings and worried parents.

I have a book about the first five years of a child's life and I read that infants of the age that my child was then should sleep approximately 16 hours a day. That brought some furrows to my brow. I didn't believe that my baby slept that much. Over the next few days, I kept a journal and noted down every time he woke up and every time he fell asleep. The results appalled me. He was sleeping around 11.5 hours at the most. He was nowhere near 16 hours a day. Something drastic had to be done!

Then I remembered that I had read something in the paper about children and sleep when I was in my ninth month. The article was about someone by the name of Anna Wahlgren. The name rang a bell, but I knew absolutely nothing about her. I had no preconceived ideas or opinions about this individual. Nor had I read any books or articles by her. I got on the net and googled her name. I got lots of hits and among the first few was a link to her homepage. 'Good,' I thought. 'She has a homepage.' There I found information about the Good-Night's-Sleep Cure, which is a cure for sleeping problems and suitable for any child over the age of four months.

My child was seven weeks, not four months. I did some research. Was it possible to use, if not the cure itself, at least some of the cure's tools to prolong a younger infant's sleep?

Yes, it was.

I introduced set times immediately. I already had a written record of my child's sleep pattern, so now I put together a schedule. 'If the boy is going to be squaring eight hours sleep a night one week from now,' I reasoned, 'that leaves another eight hours that he is going to have to sleep during the day.' After further consideration and several sheets of paper, I had a preliminary sleep schedule ready.

This got a lot of laughs when my friends found out. 'It will never work!' some said. 'Lots of luck!' said others with a grin. I took the criticism in my stride. 'Now I'm taking over,' I thought to myself. 'I have been following my child's every move for seven weeks, and he has no idea!'

After his first day on a fixed schedule, the little lad slept four hours at a stretch during the night. He woke up for one night feeding – and promptly slept another four hours. We now had a happy infant who had gotten enough sleep. Whining and crying gave way to smiles and then to happy babbling.

Did this kid cry when mother laid down the law on when he was going to eat and when he was going to sleep? No, he didn't.

For the first few days, I let him take his naps in the baby carriage. Obviously, there were times when I put down a little guy who was wide-awake. He looked at me with eyes that were wondering what on earth I thought I was doing. 'Am I supposed to sleep now?' The answer in the form of a vigorous rocking of the carriage was, 'You got it pal.' And very soon his eyes rolled up and his lids came down. Then I stopped rocking and went on my way. He would have to fall asleep himself. And he did. Without crying.

No system is perfect unfortunately. There were of course times when he woke up in the middle of a nap anything but rested. We might have company at such times. Did I get some dirty looks! 'Why doesn't she pick the baby up?' 'What's with all the carriage rocking?' 'If the kid quiets down so much when she rocks him, why doesn't she do it until he's sound asleep?' And on and on, forever and ever, amen. (Then again, it's perfectly possible that this monologue was all in my head and my curious guests were completely innocent...)

With the help of Anna Wahlgren's strategy, I successively prolonged my child's sleep. I didn't have to put a sobbing little boy to bed. On the contrary, he would start to nod off during the last evening feeding. Would I have time to put him down before he was sound asleep? When he went down for the night, he got his good-night jingle. One repeat performance, a little quieter this time, and he was off to dreamland.

Did he never wake up in the middle of the night? Of course he did. The pre-dawn hours between four and six were a little chaotic for a few weeks. I would jump out of bed and rock him (he slept in the baby carriage, even at night) countless times during 'the hour of the wolf'. During this period, I would discuss the existence or non-existence of the Wolf with other mothers (who were applying the cure) on Anna Wahlgren's forum.

Finally the night came when my son slept the whole night without waking up once. And he did it all by himself.

We have had twelve-hour nights since he was four months old. All of us, my little boy most of all, are ecstatic about this. He is one happy baby. If he does happen to wake up, he gets his good night jingle and silence descends. He has fallen back to sleep.

Newborns know that their chances of surviving on their own are nil. They cannot feed themselves, warm themselves or defend themselves against wild animals. Newborn's helplessness – their powerlessness – is total.

On the other side of the scale is the instinct to survive, which is the strongest instinct human beings have.

There can be only one result: survival anxiety. Newborn children want to survive and have to survive, but they are convinced that they are going to die.

It is precisely this survival anxiety that the 'flock' into which the child has been born must do everything in its power to eliminate.

I know that you, all of you who are now holding this book in your hands, have done everything in your power to get your children to sleep. Yet, you have not succeeded. Instead, your children's sleep problems are getting worse.

You will soon understand why.

If you are caring for an infant or a very young child, words won't get you very far. Your actions must speak for themselves. It is a question of constantly reassuring a child, through your actions, that he or she will survive.

You are in effect saying: 'You will survive. We will make sure of it. We are looking out for your interests. You can, in peace and quiet, devote yourself to living, growing and developing. And as a nice little dividend on the side, you can have fun while you're doing it! The wolves aren't coming for you. You can rest easy.'

Children's basic needs must be satisfied. Their needs are exactly the same as yours: sufficient food at somewhat regular intervals, sufficient sleep at somewhat regular intervals, clothes on their backs and a roof over their heads, a place on earth that they can call home, and people with whom they can stand shoulder to shoulder in the collective struggle for survival.

Young children cannot provide any of these things for themselves. Adults, who have mastered the art of survival, must step up to the plate and deliver.

Just as you, a mother or a father, make it possible for your young child to eat by feeding her (let's say it's a little girl), so must you make it possible for your child to sleep by ensuring that she is all safe, protected from the wolf in all its forms.

You believe you have tried everything. But there is still something wrong, since your child is not sleeping. If all the measures you have taken, night after night, to get your child to sleep were the right ones, your little one would be sleeping soundly.

The bitter truth is that, in spite of all your good intentions, you have exacerbated your child's survival anxiety rather than eliminating it.

Every time you pick your child up from the bed at night, you are adding fuel to the fire. You are, through your actions, saying that the world is just as unpredictable and dangerous as your child, in her worst moments of survival anxiety, fears it is. You are offering the child protection in your anxious embrace, thereby sending the message that your child's life is in mortal danger without such protection.

An infant is no more convinced that a bed is a safe place than you would be convinced that a tent was a safe place if you were camping out on the savannah and a pride of lions was sniffing at the tent flap – and you are an adult.

'Am I really supposed to be lying here all by myself?' your child screams from her bed. 'Isn't it dangerous? Won't the wolf come and get me?'

If your answer to your child's questions – and the only way newborns can ask questions is to scream – is to pick her up from her bed, offer her the protection of your body, comfort her and carry her, you are in effect *saving* your child. Through your actions you are shouting, 'No, you can't possibly lie here! Your bed is a death trap! We have to get you somewhere safe!'

Even if your child allows herself to be temporarily comforted in your arms, the answer you have given is hardly comforting in the long run.

Furthermore, it isn't true. Your child's bed *isn't* dangerous. The wolf *isn't* there.

Your child will not accept such a misleading answer because no human being, big or small, has the strength to live in constant fear of her life. No one who thinks she might not survive from one day to the next can sleep well at night.

That is why your child wakes up, screams and asks questions night after night, more and more obstinately.

What your little one wants is reassurance in the true sense of the word. The message she wants to hear is, 'You can sleep safe and secure. We are watching over you. We know the danger and we will keep it at bay. Your survival is guaranteed.'

Little Elliott's mother writes:
It's so much fun being with a happy baby!
We did the cure in January, when Elliott was just over six months old. It went

very well. Surpassed all our expectations! He was already sleeping twelve hours by the third night. Then we had a week or two when we had to contend with some fussing during the pre-dawn hours or an early start to the day, but it was easy to fix.

And that's the point. It's so easy! It's as though Elliott simply asked for help to sleep and then gratefully accepted the new routines.

He has always been a strong, well-built little guy, but now his development has exploded. He was crawling when he was just over seven months and now he is up and walking with his little walker at only ten months.

He has been down with a cold once, but it didn't disturb his nocturnal sleep. And he has gotten two new teeth without even a hint of sleep problems.

Watching how our son responded so quickly to the Good-Night's-Sleep Cure has been a bewildering experience. Suddenly, there are no limits. I have seen the light! Now I know how you care for and raise children!

Another mother confirms her child's relief:

A whole year of blissful nocturnal sleep for our little (nowadays big!) boy. One year and two nights ago, we started the Good-Night's-Sleep Cure for our then four-month-old son. And the results were nothing short of miraculous. Those 'cry nights' were soon but a distant memory.

Who would have imagined that a day would come when he would stretch out his arms towards the bed and laugh before he dropped off?

Yet another testimonial from a mother:

We gave our son the cure when he was just over five months old. We had been thinking about it for a while but were hesitant about taking the plunge.

Our son slept very badly. He would doze off at my breast or while I rocked the cradle, but he would wake up constantly. There always seemed to be something bothering him. I would nurse him, carry him around and try to lull him back to sleep, but all he did was scream. At five in the morning my husband would spell me so I could grab a couple of hours sleep.

We felt that the situation simply wasn't sustainable. My husband and I were *tired and crabby. Our son was tired and whiny, and his poor older sister was caught in the middle.*

At that time, Anna's parent forum wasn't available, but her Cheat Sheet was. Which we copied and read. And read again!

On a long weekend, we started the cure. And our son seemed to heave a sigh of relief and promptly went to sleep. The jingle was just the ticket. Pure magic!

It took around five weeks for the night and the pre-dawn hours to merge smoothly, but it was nothing we couldn't handle. We were a whole new family. The summer was fabulous, just as it should be with two young children!

This coming May, it will be two years since we started the cure and, by and large, our son has slept very well. There were times when he would wake up early, but thanks to stubborn use of the jingle, they have passed. Sometimes persistent illnesses caused problems, but with the cure's strategies and all the advice from the forum, we were soon back on track.

Today, he sleeps 11–12 hours a night and 1.5 to 2 hours in the middle of the day. We are eternally grateful!

Our only regret is that we didn't start the cure sooner.

The wolf exists. It cannot be denied or comforted away. It must be held at bay proactively and continuously.

We adults, who know the drill, do it all the time. It was to keep wild animals away that human beings first built dwellings.

Every day and every night, you and I and all the other people on the planet take a range of measures to ensure that we do not fall prey to the wolf in one of its forms. We look both ways before we cross the street. We check that our doors are locked before we go to bed. We install smoke alarms in our houses. We disconnect electrical appliances and make sure the stove is off before we leave our homes. We lock, turn on the alarm system and shut the wolf out with all the means at our disposal.

We know what can happen. Danger always threatens. We spare no effort to protect ourselves.

Children want to be reassured that the wolf won't come for them. Children want to be reassured that no danger threatens. Children want to sleep just as soundly as you do once you have blown out the candles, checked that the smoke detector is in good working order, closed the windows on the ground floor and locked the front door carefully.

You don't want to have to worry about the house catching fire while you are asleep or about an intruder breaking in and killing you in your bed. You want to sleep peacefully.

Your young child does too.

Young children cannot take any security precautions. Your young child can do absolutely nothing to make sure the wolf stays on the right side of the door. Only you, an adult skilled in the art of survival, can do that.

Therefore, the fundamental principle on which the *Good-Night's-Sleep Cure* rests is this: *young children are to be calmed where they are lying.*

Their cries are questions, not expressions of discontent.

'Is the wolf going to come and get me?' cries the child.

Your answer, in the form of instant action, is truthful, calm and reassuring:

'I am looking out for your interests. I will see to it that the wolf doesn't come for you. You can sleep in peace. You can feel completely safe. I am standing between you and the wolf. Nothing bad is going to happen to you.'

The following is a report from Lisa's mom:
It is evening on night 13 of the cure for Lisa, six months. I have been sitting on the sofa since Lisa fell asleep. I came to think of something that Anna wrote, which those of you who have given your child the cure will surely recognize: 'So what are you going to do with all that free time?'

That is my problem right now!

Those words struck me as almost malicious the first time I read them, which wasn't that long ago. I was dizzy from exhaustion, my body was a mass of pins and needles, my ears were ringing and my eyes were filled with tears after another night in hell.

I was constantly being woken up by Lisa's screams and pacifier terror. Lisa would wake up between 5 and 17 times a night at regular intervals, so I was never able to sleep more than two hours at a stretch at most. Lisa's dad even took her to work with him. I was beside myself that last morning, just before we started the cure.

What a difference! Last night, the twelfth night of the cure, Lisa slept from 7.40 in the evening to 7.25 this morning – a touch under 12 hours of continuous sleep – without so much as a peep out of her. When I went into her room this morning, she was lying in her crib, happy as a clam and deep in conversation with one of her cuddly toy friends, and obviously secure in her bed and herself!

I slept continuously from 10.00 in the evening until 7.00 in the morning. I didn't feel that I had to turn in at the same time she did so that I could get a few more hours in bed. I actually sat up and watched some TV. Little things like that are such luxuries.

I had almost forgotten how DIVINE it feels to wake up in the morning after an unbroken night's sleep... It felt as though I had woken up in another body. Just the knowledge that I will in all probability be able to sleep well enables me to relax.

The road has been hard at times to be sure, but the fabulous results make the effort more than worth it!

I also feel that I have gotten to know Lisa so much better during this cure. We have really talked to each other these last few nights, she with her questions, protests and reactions, I with my jingles and different tones of voice. I have gotten much better at really hearing her and figuring out what she is actually saying, even during the day, now that the pacifier isn't in the way and she is allowed to express herself!

Who was it that said, 'Young children should be enjoyed – and enjoy themselves'...? That is just how things feel now. And I should add that young children should be able to enjoy a happy, playful mom and not have to put up with someone who just wants to go to bed and sleep all the time!

We hope that this happy situation will continue, and I am convinced it will because now I know what to do if there is a crisis. I am calm and at the same time overjoyed!

I would also like to say that if you are about to start this cure, prepare your surroundings and get all the help you can! Having my sister around, cheering me on from the mattress the first two nights gave me a real boost, since obviously I was a little unsure of myself at the beginning. The fact that my parents were able to take Lisa out during the first few days, so that I could get a little sleep in preparation for the night to come, was also enormously helpful.

A big thank you to all of you out there on the forum for your help. Special thanks to you, Anna! If anyone deserves a Nobel Prize, it's you. I have my life back!

PS. Am I the only one who thinks that children's clinics should be pushing the Good-Night's-Sleep Cure? I didn't get much support at that end.

I think they get hung up on laying children on their stomachs, which is of course what infants prefer, whether they are asleep or awake, but which doctors advise against if the children are being put down to sleep. I was a little doubtful too at one point, but every morning without exception I have found Lisa on her back, even though she started the night on her stomach. With the help of this cure, she would sleep well standing on her head! It isn't the position that enables her to sleep well and, above all, fall asleep by herself (which was the most important thing for us), but the jingles, which convince her that we are at the door keeping the wolf away. She feels secure. It's that simple.

She knows what the rules are. She knows how she fits in. She gets the same reassuring treatment every evening and night. The fact that I had to cure my own need to be in control, as well as a severe case of mommy-to-the-rescue syndrome, and accept that she actually slept better undisturbed in her own room than she did in our bed is a saga in itself!

Perhaps a look at my nocturnal notes will perk up anyone who is in the middle of the cure. Here they are:

Night 1
She fell asleep after 40 minutes of buffing. Woke up eight times and got buffing and jingles. Sounded angry but not sad. Fell asleep several times on her own. Talked happily to herself towards morning.

Night 2
Fell asleep with buffing + jingle in five minutes. No protests. Bone tired. Woke up five times. Took 20 minutes to get her back to sleep around 4. An angry young lady.

Night 3

Fell asleep with buffing and jingles in ten minutes. No protests. Woke up at 10.30, got a quiet little jingle, fell asleep and then managed the WHOLE night by herself! Could hear her whimper the odd time, but she seemed to sleep more deeply than she ever had before. Was on cloud nine today and wanted to shout 'Anna for President' from the rooftops! Almost button-holed a pregnant woman at the grocery store to give her some preparatory tips.

Night 4

Fell asleep without protest in five minutes with a jingle and corrective positioning. Woke up eight times again at intervals evenly distributed over the night. Very angry at the beginning, but more compliant each time until 6.00 a.m., when she got angry again and stayed that way until morning. Will she hit her stride tonight?

Night 5

Out like a light in no time. Not so much as a peep after the jingle and corrective positioning. Jingles at 9.30 and 11.00. Woke up 4 times but fell back to sleep by herself.

Night 6

Fell asleep in 15 minutes. A little whiny. Was putting her on her stomach around 8.00 and happened to wake her. She was sad, but she fell back to sleep after three jingles. Woke up at 3.50 but fell asleep again by herself. Jingle at 5.35. Between 6 and 7 little whimpers and peeps, but she quieted down before I felt it was necessary to intervene. Have to make morning 7.15 since she starts to get livelier then.

Night 7

Fell asleep in 10–15 minutes. Happy. Needed jingles 4.30 and 6. 6.15–6.45. Tough half hour with one ticked-off, apparently alert kid. Firm jingles, had to go in and buff twice. Silence at last! Whew! Morning at 7.25. Didn't exactly feel my best this morning. Neither did Lisa.

Night 8

Fell asleep in 10 minutes. Happy. We had guests and there was a little more activity than normal. I was a little nervous that it would disturb her, but no problems there. She woke up but fell back to sleep by herself at 4 and 5. At 6 I had to give her a jingle. Whimpered a little from time to time between 6 and 7.15. When I went in at 7.25, she was awake and playing contentedly with her toy friend. Such a cutie!

Night 9

Fell asleep in 15 minutes. Happy. Lay in her bed and talked to herself (or with her toy friend?). 4.35, 5.50 and 6 jingles required. Between 6 and 7 she whimpered some. At 7.25 it's good morning. Lisa was playing with her toy friend.

Night 10

Asleep in 10 minutes. Happy. 1.30 upset, didn't listen to the jingle. Went in and put her on her stomach. She relaxed and I went out and jingled gently. Half awake between 6 and 7. A few sounds, a little coughing. Upset at 7. I tried jingles for about 10 minutes, but no dice. During a silent interlude, went in and it was good morning.

Night 11

Fell asleep in about ten minutes as usual. Lay there and talked happily to herself. Woke up at 3 but fell back to sleep by herself. Needed help at 4.20, 6.10, 6.30 and 6.55 with jingles. Waited. On tenterhooks because I was afraid she would get worked up before I had time to go in... Was patient until 7.20, when I went in for a happy good morning reunion.

Night 12

Asleep in 10 minutes. Happy. Was woken up by her dad's alarm clock at 7!!! Was frightened at first. Was she still alive? Then heard her talking in her room.

Went in at 7.25. She was deep in conversation with her toy friend and didn't notice me at first. Then the cutest little smile lit up her face.

A start like that to the day is such pure joy!

CHILDREN AND SLEEP

Tomorrow my little prince turns three. I look back and think how fantastic my life suddenly became that mid-summer afternoon three years ago.

But it hasn't been all *champagne and caviar. I wanted nothing more than to be a really great mother, and my son couldn't have been more loved or longed for. He should have been as content and inwardly harmonious as it is possible for a baby to be. But all he did was cry and scream. He never slept more than 45 minutes at a stretch. Max!*

I hung on for four and a half months, and then I broke down. I took my son home from parents' day at play school with tears streaming down my cheeks. I was a lousy mother. Why else would he be so miserable all the time?

Then I got a tip about Anna's forum. I read extensively, asked a lot of questions and got to work. Three days later, my boy was sleeping the whole night plus taking his naps during the day! Suddenly, I had a son who was cheerful, content and curious about the world. He would lie there on his blanket pleased as punch with everything. A week later at play school, people commented on how we had both changed.

Today he is one happy boy, good-humored, only moderately defiant at his low points, and unbearably charming. And that's according to other people!

We can go on trips and sleep anywhere. He sleeps like a log with that internal eat-and-sleep clock of his, no matter where we are.

So, on his third birthday, I want to thank you for being there and having the strength to help all of us who couldn't figure things out by ourselves.

His little sister came along six months ago. She probably has you, Anna to thank for her existence. We would never have considered bringing another child into the world if you hadn't helped us find our feet.

Big hugs from all of us,
Helen, who has the world's greatest family.

A human cub is a helpless being for a very long time. Every minute, every hour, every day and every night for many years – longer than any other mammal – she is dependent on her surroundings for the care and protection that she cannot provide for herself.

We were all little once. Once upon a time, you too knew that you would surely die if no one took care of you. We have all been plagued by survival anxiety. We have all had to look the wolf, its teeth bared, in the eye.

Newborns are instinctively aware of their helpless vulnerability. What little experience they do have tells them that life is fragile. They must emerge from the womb, where they were never hungry, never had to breathe, never were cold and never knew danger. They had to leave the womb behind them because suddenly the food and the oxygen were cut off.

They were not born yearning to know their mothers or curious about their fathers. They were born out of the jaws of death, tormented by survival anxiety.

Caught in the vice of survival anxiety, they drew their first breath, which they then exhaled in the form of a scream. They had never breathed before.

Naturally, they cannot grasp that breathing means that the air they are drawing into their lungs will oxygenate their blood, thus making it possible for them to go on living. They breathe because they *have to* breathe.

Nor do they understand that sucking, which they are hardwired to do, means that the liquid they take into their mouths and swallow will nourish them and save their lives. They suck because they have to. The equation *food in mouth = full stomach = satisfied hunger = sense of well being = alleviated survival anxiety* does not exist for them.

This equation is eventually revealed through experience, just as breathing one day becomes automatic. But that day is still a long way off.

Some children are born with more acute survival anxiety than others, just as there is usually a chick in a bird's nest who cries more lustily than the others and manages to pinch the fattest worms from the beaks of their less robust siblings.

Baby birds don't have colic. And neither do baby humans.

No child has ever been born with colic.

The moment survival anxiety is alleviated – with food, more food, and still more food – 'colic', 'upset stomach' – and all the other 'ailments' that are usually invoked to explain the desperate crying of newborns – promptly vanish.

Colic is unalleviated survival anxiety.

For infants to dare believe that life will continue tomorrow, food, more food, and still more food is not the only requirement. They also need the *strength* to live. They need the strength to enjoy the environment into which they have been born.

They must have the strength to derive pleasure from the *joie de vivre* and the life force that characterize and guide the human instinct to survive.

They can't do that without sleep, sufficient sleep, and even a little more sleep.

How much sleep do children need?

At one month: 16.5 hours per 24-hour period
At two months: 16/24
At three and four months: 15.5/24
At five and six months: 15/24
At seven and eight months: 14.5/24
At nine, ten and eleven months: 14/24
At twelve months to two years: 13.5/24
Years three and four: 13/24
Years five and six: 12.5/24
Years seven to eleven: 12/24

A newborn's sleep can be likened to oblivion. An infant simply passes out any time, anywhere. Anyone who has tried to wake a newborn knows that it is virtually impossible.

When newborns fall asleep, it is as though a candle has been blown out. They sink into a merciful slumber, which for a while – often for several hours – insulates them from the trauma of birth as well as survival anxiety.

In the womb, there was no hunger, no eating, no struggle to breathe, no cold, and no fatigue. Life was simply a matter of growing and playing in a familiar environment. This secure existence was abruptly terminated. Life literally hung by a thread – the umbilical cord – which had hitherto provided both sustenance and oxygen. And this thread was cut.

This secure life was replaced by something else and it was anything but secure.

'Young children take as much sleep as they need,' all you new parents have no doubt been told. 'It's not something you have to worry about. Just let your baby decide!'

This holds true for newborns, who sleep like the dead. And it certainly holds true for unborn children!

However, the newborn period is brief. It lasts for the first two weeks of life and sometimes the first half of the third.

At this point, something I call *the true birth* occurs. Your child, who has recovered from the traumatic shock of birth and all that it entailed, will now begin to turn outward in every sense of the word, and a stubborn struggle for social participation will ensue.

From the true birth on, few if any children take the sleep they need all by themselves.

It isn't something we can demand of them.

Nor can we demand that they take the food they need all by themselves.

You don't expect your baby to be able to point to the fridge and whimper when hunger sets in. Nor do you expect her to pull off your sweater, loosen your bra, and pull out your breast.

You make it possible for your baby to eat. You serve the food. You single-mindedly press food upon your baby because you know that she needs nourishment.

You can't eat for your child. But what you can and must do, several times a day, is to give your baby the prerequisites to nourish herself.

I think you would have been very surprised if a pediatrician or a nurse at your local children's clinic had said, 'Babies take the food they need all by themselves. It's nothing you have to worry about. Just let your child decide!'

Infants can neither see to their own sustenance, nor achieve that state of inner peace that is required for them to be able to – or to dare – to sleep peacefully, secure in themselves.

They cannot ensure their own survival.

They cannot keep the wolf at bay.

Little Belinda's mother writes:
We often think back to that day at the beginning of the summer when we decided to give our daughter the cure. She was five months old at the time. Now she is a year old and a little Sleeping Beauty.

Today we were at the children's clinic for a vaccination and the nurse anxiously asked us, 'How is she sleeping? Is everything alright?'

When I replied that she was sleeping twelve hours a night and two hours during the day, she looked astonished and asked where you could order kids like that.

I told her that all she had to do was call Anna Wahlgren.

With the advent of the true birth, a new kind of crying comes into the picture. If nine out of ten cries from an infant are expressions of survival anxiety that can be stilled with food, more food, and still more food, the tenth is an expression of overtiredness.

The world forces its way in. Hundreds of thousands of impressions and stimuli bombard a young child every day.

A three-week-old cannot shut out a world that very often simply becomes too much to bear. Infants cannot take mental holidays the way adults can.

After the true birth, infants can no longer retreat into merciful oblivion. They need help to find peace.

The sleep they do get is very different from that of a newborn. It is more normal, more like adult sleep. It renews and refreshes. It gives all a newborn's senses, which operate at full throttle every waking second, a wholesome and vitally necessary time out.

There is no reason to feel sorry for a young child who is able to sleep. It is an advantage that should be given to all young children and all beings of flesh and blood for that matter.

And your little one is made of the same stuff that you are.

Never before has children's need for a sound, undisturbed, continuous night's sleep been called into question as it is today – but that is another, very tragic, story.

A first-time mother writes:

I read 'For the Love of Children' as a teenager and I couldn't wait to have kids. It all sounded so easy!

Thankfully, God waited fifteen years before answering my prayers. The fourteen-year-old me was not as ready for motherhood as she thought, but Anna's tips stayed with me.

Routines, social participation and simple bedtime rituals all combined brilliantly. My daughter hardly ever cried and she developed at break-neck speed.

Then things got difficult. When she began to cry at bedtime and during the night, I was caught off guard. I began to cradle her in my arms and lull her to sleep with a bottle of formula. During the night, I would be running in and out of her room trying to pat her back to sleep. Once or twice a night was no problem, but her wakeful periods got longer and more frequent, and life soon became unbearable.

I thought that giving her the whole Good-Night's-Sleep Cure *was an over-reaction. She could sleep after all!*

One evening I read about what the Cure advises in case of small 'relapses' or new questions: a jingle, let the reaction fade into silence, and jingle again when she falls silent or she becomes unhappy and wants her question answered again.

Bingo! I put her to bed when she was still awake, jingled and left the room. I waited outside the door for her to finish reacting. And guess what happened! She fell asleep all by herself after three minutes of complaining and a confirmation jingle. She only woke up once that night. The following evening she was asleep in less than a minute and she slept right through the night.

Now, four weeks later, she sometimes wakes up and cries, but she is content with an answering jingle (instead of an hour of patting in her crib which meant a sore back for me and frustration for both of us), and such episodes are become more and more infrequent.

Every evening at 7.00, when I put her down, she is wakeful and happy. She snuggles into her pillow and falls asleep by herself after I have left. She has discovered how good it feels to sleep. Going to bed takes no longer than the jingle itself.

In the mornings, I make sure that she doesn't need to call out to me, and more often than not I have to wake a dozy little baby at 7.00 a.m.

Do I need to tell you that my daughter and the rest of the family are pleased over this turn of events? I am amazed and I feel a little sheepish!

Every child is born with a magic wand in her hand. Nature has pulled out all the stops to ensure that the child survives.

From the moment the child is born, the two parents, who have been preparing during nine months of pregnancy, stand ready to shoulder the responsibility for another human being's well being 24 hours a day. They feel a *will* to love, which they would scarcely feel for a kid that was dumped in their front hall with a note telling them to provide for this child day and night for a couple of decades.

Mother Nature had prepared the ground. The readiness on the part of the parents is total.

But infants don't know this when they are born. They have just emerged from the jaws of death into the light.

The birth itself is an appalling experience. The baby has been rotated down through a birth canal so narrow that the two halves of her skull sometimes overlap under the pressure before her face is pried up and out.

Immediately thereafter, her lungs are put to work, lungs that have never known air.

The child takes in oxygen and forces out her first breath in the form of a scream. Her own scream is also unknown to her.

Everything is unknown and terrifying, the sounds, the light, the cold – the temperature difference is a brutal fifteen degrees – and the whole world is new.

It is not hard to understand that this unknown world must seem full of mortal danger to a newborn.

It is impossible to explain to a newborn that everything will be all right. It is impossible to explain that her survival is guaranteed. It is impossible to reassure her that the wolf is not waiting to pounce. It is impossible to tell her that there is no risk and that she will not freeze to death, starve to death or be left to her fate in the forest.

Words are useless. The adults must give guarantees of survival through their actions.

First and foremost, the child must have food. Food and physical warmth. Food and human warmth. Food and protection from the wolf. Food and merciful, restful sleep.

With the exception of brand-new arrivals, who sleep the sleep of the dead, infants cannot take the sleep they need for themselves.

The sequence *feel tired-lie down-be quiet-fall asleep-wake up feeling better* doesn't exist for them.

They fear for their lives. 'Am I going to go under?'

They fear the wolf, which in the Western tradition symbolizes everything that poses a threat to life and limb.

In the grip of survival anxiety as they are, they scream. They are asking for security. They are asking for help to be at peace.

So that they dare to sleep peacefully, they need help, just as they need help with the breast, the bottle, the Pablum and the purée to be able to eat.

Infants can no more take the food they need all by themselves than they can take the sleep they need.

A mother reflects:
I was with my little guy at an infant massage course last Tuesday.

The instructor asked us why we were taking the course. Seven out of ten people said that they had come because of their children's stomach problems or 'colic'.

I looked at these children. Their eyes were red. Their skin was pale. Some of them cried incessantly, in spite of the fact that 'all kids love massage' (except for the over-tired ones maybe), while others just lay there and stared.

I got the urge to take all these kids home and feed them, rock them, and buff them to peaceful headspace until my arms fell off. It was so obvious that these kids were suffering from food and sleep deprivation!

'When your child begins to cry at 6.00 p.m. sharp and refuses to stop until 2.00 in the morning' said the instructor, 'here's what you do. No feeding. Carry your child around in your arms. That helps sometimes. Massage. Go for a drive. Avoid dairy and grain products if you are breastfeeding. These problems usually don't last for longer than three months!'

Dear instructor, sorry to burst your bubble, but haven't you forgotten something? Two important needs that all human beings have? Sleep for example? Not to mention food in large quantities?

It just made me want to scream. Massage is lovely, but it doesn't cure survival anxiety.

My goal is to see to it that the *Good-Night's-Sleep Cure* replaces and consigns to oblivion a technique that goes under such names as the Five Minute Method, the Cry-It-Out Method, or the Controlled Crying Method as it is known internationally.

'Why?' you may be wondering. 'Isn't it much simpler to let an infant scream herself to sleep for a few nights until she figures out that she might just as well sleep?'

Isn't what you have read so far about the *Good-Night's-Sleep Cure* far more difficult than putting up with a little crying? You have to make up a schedule for 'rocking', 'buffing' and 'jingling'. Why can't you just leave every-thing to the child?

To understand the big difference between the Controlled Crying Method and the *Good-Night's-Sleep Cure*, you have to understand the wolf analogy. You have to be able to understand survival anxiety from your child's point of view, anxiety that you yourself experienced once upon a time.

Unlike the Controlled Crying Method, the *Good-Night's-Sleep Cure* places responsibility on the parents.

It is the adults who must help their child find peace.

It is the adults who must do battle with the wolf – survival anxiety – force him to turn tail and lock him out.

It is the adults who must guarantee their child's survival and much more besides. They must guarantee a good life, a secure life with good sleep, peaceful sleep, sufficient sleep and blissful sleep, sleep that their baby will soon joyously take, secure enough in herself to both dare and desire to sleep that well.

The principle underlying the Controlled Crying Method has its roots in the United States in the 1940s. It stipulates that infants shall cry themselves to sleep, while the parents look in on them every five minutes (at best) and let the infants know that the parents are there.

This method makes the children responsible for calming themselves down as best they can. It demands strong nerves on the part of the parents, who are expected to suppress their protective instincts, which tell them to whisk their distressed offspring to safety.

It is true enough that the little ones fall asleep sooner or later, since their crying eventually leads to resignation and exhaustion. Consequently, the Controlled Crying Method does work – provided that the parents are resilient enough to justify their passivity in the face of their child's more or less hysterical despair.

However, the Controlled Crying Method has grave shortcomings.

1. The unanswered cries inevitably result in feelings of abandonment. For a young child who cannot survive on her own, abandonment equals a death sentence.

2. Sleep that is the result of resignation, despair and mental exhaustion is seldom particularly refreshing. That goes for all of us.
3. The vast majority of children that are 'cured' by the Controlled Crying Method sleep far too little. The parents have to exhaust them before putting them to bed. Understandably enough, everyone wants to avoid hours of crying.
4. Sleep that children neither want nor enjoy is easily disrupted by the least bit of stress, such as teething or colds. The results obtained through the use of the Controlled Crying Method are therefore seldom permanent. The Method has to be applied again and again.

The *Good-Night's-Sleep Cure*, on the other hand, ensures that young children's questions never go unanswered. The cries that express their fear for their lives, their fear of the wolf, their anxiety over their own indisputable helplessness must never go unanswered.

In my opinion, young children should not cry at all.

They do anyway, of course, but the myriad of questions they ask during the first evening of the *Good-Night's-Sleep Cure* should be met with immediate and, in the true sense of the word, *satisfying* answers – even if the first answer takes a laborious 20–45 minutes to get across to an infant who has never slept well (or at all for that matter).

Young children can be in a lousy mood, they can be angry and generally react less than nobly, but in my world infants and young children should *not* be distressed or unhappy.

Young children should never be permitted to feel that they have been abandoned for a single second.

A young mother writes:
We followed the instructions in 'For the Love of Children' to the letter. We stuffed him to the gills and gradually rocked away the night feedings.

And oh how everyone laughed.

'A four-month-old sleeping 12 hours a night! Yeah, right! Lots of luck!'

But then he turned four months and he really did sleep 12 hours a night.

'Yeah, but wait a while. As soon as he gets a cold or a new tooth, that'll be the end of that! You've just been lucky so far.'

And he did get a cold. And stomach flu. And two new teeth. Now the little guy has learned to crawl and stand. And he is still sleeping his 12 hours a night.

We have had to jingle the odd time, but he falls back to sleep immediately.

I'm sure you can guess how much I like throwing that in the faces of all the sceptics!

THE SAFARI – AN ALLEGORY

Imagine you are on safari. You have been dreaming about going on safari for several years. Now you are doing it!

You are in the middle of no man's land. It's only your first day and you have already seen scores of wild animals. Early tomorrow morning, you are going bird watching. You are part of a small group that is eagerly seeking breathtaking close encounters with Nature.

And your guide is fabulous. He is knowledgeable and confident, and he adores his work. You have complete confidence in him. He has porters, cooks, scouts and all manner of experts to help him. This is truly a world-class operation!

From day one, you have been very professionally looked after.

This enterprise is not cheap, but it's worth every penny. It has surpassed your wildest expectations!

You make camp and night falls. You enjoy a hearty dinner around the campfire. The conversation is exhilarating. You even got to see a lion earlier in the day. A large male, close enough to touch, was indolently stretched out in the sun. What an experience! Your traveling companions are as excited as you are.

You are given your own tent to sleep in out there in the bush. There are one-person tents for solitary sojourners, and you appreciate that. You want to be left in peace with no disturbances. It makes for a better night's sleep.

The guide provides you with a blanket and a pillow, and wishes you good night. Before he goes, he takes you aside and gives you a friendly word of warning. 'Make sure you stay on your cot during the night. Scorpions and poisonous spiders sometimes get into the tents.'

You scramble up onto your cot and try to draw your knees up to your chin.

No need to be nervous, you tell yourself. It has been a long, somewhat overwhelming day. Your poor brain has been bombarded with new impressions, and you are tired. You're dying to sleep.

You lie there in the dark, vaguely aware of the light from the campfire, listening to the jungle's nocturnal symphony. Your eyelids feel heavy.

But what was that? What was that sound? Wasn't that a lion roaring right outside your tent?

You sit bolt upright on your cot. There's a lion out there! You heard it roar! And there it is again! A lion is roaring for all he is worth right outside your tent!

Your heart is pounding. Frozen with fear, you stare into the darkness towards the entrance to the tent. The material is flimsy. Thin canvas. It offers no protection. You realize in horror how easy it would be for the lion to rip through the tent flap and pounce on you in the darkness.

Oh God, it's roaring again! Wasn't it closer this time? Your heart is beating so loudly it all but drowns out your terrified thoughts.

You try to pull yourself together. You have to do something. But what? You are all alone in this pathetic little tent out in the middle of nowhere, and you won't have a chance if the lion decides to attack.

The roaring again! You are awash in icy sweat.

You don't scream. You are an adult after all, and even if you have never been this petrified in your life, you are going to conduct yourself with decorum.

You clear your throat nervously.

'Hello!' you cry timidly towards the tent flap. 'Is anyone there? Hello...?'

What an indescribable relief! The tent flaps part and in the campfire's feeble light, you see the barrel of a rifle. And who is holding the gun? Your guide, your wonderful, splendid, glorious guide!

Now you see him clearly, and he is truly a sight for sore eyes.

'No problem,' he says with a reassuring smile. 'I'm standing guard out here. You can rest easy.'

You are so relieved, you want to throw your arms around him. But there's that business with the scorpions...

'I thought I heard a lion,' you manage to gasp.

'No lion would dare get this close,' the guide reassures you. 'And if one were stupid enough to try, he'd only do it once, believe you me.'

He leaves. The tent flaps close. Reassured, you lie down again. Your heart slowly descends from your throat and assumes its customary position. You fall into a sound sleep.

But what was that? You heard it again.

You sit up on the bunk with a start, wide-awake. Your heart is going like a jackhammer. Now you hear not just one, but *several* lions. There are at least three of them out there roaring like it's going out of style. You could swear that there is one on each side of the tent and one behind you.

How long have you been asleep? You don't know. If only this were a nightmare, but no such luck. You can see the lions skulking around the tent, casting their ominous shadows on the canvas. They are all around you! Their roaring engulfs you in the dark jungle night.

Frantically, you try to get a grip on yourself. The sweat trickles down your face, your heart pounds. You try to think...

The guide said that he would stand guard. He told you that you could rest easy. If the lions came, he would take care of them. He promised.

But what if he doesn't stay at his post? The guide needs to sleep too, doesn't he? What if he doesn't hear the lions? Maybe he has a girlfriend out here in the bush somewhere and he is sleeping with her in some distant tent. He might not have the faintest inkling that your life is hanging in the balance!

Now the lions are roaring again. You are convinced that one of them, or two, or maybe all three are going to storm the tent at any moment, rip it to shreds and sink their blood-thirsty fangs into your flesh. They are going to tear you limb from limb!

'Hello!' you whimper again, and now you sound every bit as terrified as you actually are. 'Hello? Is anyone there? Hellooo?'

Do you dare hope for the same wonderful sight as last time? No, you don't! The lions are roaring in the darkness. Can the guide hear them, even if he is standing just outside? Maybe they've got him too!

But thank the Lord, there he is!

The gun barrel parts the tent flaps and the guide enters. He stands before you, large and confident, rifle at the ready.

'There's no danger,' he assures you. 'I'm here. You can rest easy.'

You would throw yourself at his feet in blissful gratitude if it weren't for the scorpions.

You're still afraid, but doesn't the roaring of the lions seem a little more distant now? Maybe they weren't as close as you thought. Maybe they weren't anywhere near the tent. You know how hard it is to judge distances in the dark. And the shadows? Maybe it was only the flames of the camp-fire playing tricks on you.

But common sense doesn't allay your fears. You are still so terrified you can hardly breathe.

'They sound awfully close,' you manage to get out.

The guide sees how frightened you are. He puts down his rifle and comes closer.

'There are several of us out there,' he says soothingly. 'No one's life is in jeopardy on this safari!'

That was what you wanted to hear. You stretch out again on your narrow cot and try to swallow the lump in your throat.

The guide looks dismayed.

'Poor you,' he says and comes a little closer. 'Were you really that scared? But you don't have to be scared. I'm here. I'm with you.'

That's the problem, you think to yourself as the lump in your throat starts to grow again. The guide *is* with you. He isn't outside the tent, his rifle at the ready. His gun is out of reach. He put it down at the entrance to the tent. He is standing beside your cot looking down at you, instead of standing guard outside.

That's hardly reassuring.

You are beginning to feel nervous. This professional guide, who radiates confidence, who is security personified, is hovering over your cot looking worried.

And now you hear the lions again! They're here! They are overrunning the camp! You can hear all three of them! And they're getting closer and closer...

Panic-stricken, you stare at the guide. Doesn't he hear them? Why doesn't he do something?

You're so terrified you're on the verge of cardiac arrest.

'Dear heart,' says the guide sympathetically. 'You're so frightened! I feel so sorry for you!'

Now he comes right up to the cot, as you lie there paralyzed with fear. He tilts his head and looks at you comfortingly.

'I can lie down you with you for a bit if you like. I can pat you.'

Pat you? You are so petrified you don't know which end is up. That's very kind of him, but... the lions are roaring outside. Three of them. Their roars are so ear splitting they might as well be inside the tent. How can the guide think that the lions will go away just because he lies down beside you and pats you?

You try to think straight. He must know what he is doing. After all, he is an experienced safari guide and he knows the bush. What would happen if your cowardly side accepted his offer to lie down beside you and pat you?

He would be lying on the side nearest the entrance to the tent. He would be the one to get eaten first if the lions were to get in. That would mean at least some protection for you.

But it would be fleeting! There would still be two more lions! One would gobble down the guide, but the other two would still be hungry. You would be easy prey. Your final hour would be delayed but not by much.

No, you don't think this lie-down-and-pat stuff is a very good idea!

The guide looks worried. Then he brightens up and comes up with another suggestion.

'We can dance! Wouldn't that be nice and soothing?'

He opens his arms invitingly to take you into his embrace for a slow waltz.

Nice and soothing? You're not too sure about that. You don't think it would be particularly soothing to put your feet down among the poisonous spiders and scorpions and dance a waltz with the guide. What's more, you don't understand how dancing around the tent is going to stop these lions from launching a deadly attack at any moment.

No, you don't think this is a good idea at all.

'Shall we have a cup of tea then?' asks the guide. 'Tea for two and a nice chat, just you and me! Wouldn't that be fun? And a cakey-wakey maybe?'

Cakey-wakey? What's with the baby talk?

The guide, the man to whom you have entrusted your life and your security is smiling so tenderly at you. He seems to really want you to have a good time there in the tent.

Out in the bush.

At night.

With lions roaring just outside.

What are you supposed to think? You wonder if you are losing your mind. You are in mortal danger, and your guide is cooing at you like you were a little baby at your mother's breast!

Just at that moment, you hear a roar that is so close you don't dare straighten your arm for fear of having your hand bitten off. Your blood runs so cold it congeals in your veins. You realize that the lion has advanced to the spot where the guide should have been standing guard.

Your nerves, already stretched to breaking point, finally snap.

'Shut up and shoot something!' you howl, abandoning any pretence of decorum. 'I paid good money for this trip and I want the security I was promised. And another thing! I want to go bird watching tomorrow, and I need my sleep! Sleep! As in unconscious! So stop bothering me! Do your frigging job! Get your butt out there and stand guard!'

'Don't you like me?' asks the guide.

'What?'

You can't believe you're hearing this. And speaking of hearing, you suddenly don't hear any lions roaring.

'I thought you liked me,' says the guide.

He looks at you as though you should be worried about *him* instead of a bunch of lions and all the other things you are so scared of. He seems to be implying that you should be feeling sorry for him because you've been so mean to him. After all he has tried to do for you, all you do is yell at him!

'What does that have to do with anything?' you say. 'This isn't about *feelings!* It's about me being able to sleep and you keeping the lions away.'

'There are no lions around here,' the guide says sulkily. 'At least no dangerous ones. At least no dangerous ones that come very close to the tent. At least no dangerous ones that come very close to the tent that you have to be afraid of. At least no dangerous ones that come very close to the tent that you have to be afraid of because they might eat you. At least...'

'Don't talk so much!' you interrupt. 'Prove it.'

You're starting to wonder if the guide and his assistants, who are supposed to function as a reliable security force after dark, are really qualified for the job. Do they really think that cooing, patting, comforting, dancing, cakey-wakeys and all this talking will guarantee the *security* of the people on this safari?

At last the guide gets the message. He picks up his gun and leaves. Finally! The tent flaps close silently behind him and you feel at peace.

The lions have fallen silent. And that is pure heaven because now you are absolutely exhausted. It won't be long before it's time to get up and go bird watching and you want to be able to keep up.

And not just keep up. You want to enjoy it!

You came along on this safari because you wanted a once-in-a-lifetime experience, not a nocturnal circus like the one you have just been through.

You stretch out on the cot fully conscious of the fact that a new threat can materialize at any time and frighten you half to death. But at least now you dare to believe that the guide is at his post, armed and at the ready.

You can sleep soundly! He is not going to hang around your cot and babble about feelings.

But what was that? Was that a gunshot?

Or was it something else, one of the myriad wilderness sounds that you don't recognize?

Or are you just imagining things?

Anyway, now you can sleep in peace and that is going be sheer ecstasy!

II.

THE GOOD-NIGHT'S-SLEEP CURE: PEACE, SECURITY, ENJOYMENT!

If and when you decide to embark on the *Good-Night's-Sleep Cure*, there are three goals that you will be working towards.

• The first is to give your infant *peace*.

• The second is to give your infant *security*.

• The third and final goal is to enable your child to *enjoy* sleeping well, a knack that will hopefully last a lifetime.

You will achieve the first goal within 96 hours after you start the cure.

You will achieve the second goal during the follow-up week.

Once you have succeeded in providing your child with peace and security, neither of which will ever be called into question by you or your child, enjoyment will come of its own accord over the following few weeks. At that point, you will have crossed the finish line. You will have implemented the *Good-Night's-Sleep Cure.*

As a result, you and your family will have a new life. Then, if not before, you will understand – and whole-heartedly agree with – what I never tire of advocating.

Young children should be enjoyed, and they should enjoy themselves!

1. PEACE

Young children should *be calmed wherever they happen to be lying.* In one of the following chapters the strategies for calming a screaming infant will be described in great detail.

Words are not enough, as you have no doubt already figured out. A hands-on approach is what's needed. The tools are physical. We have touched upon them briefly: rocking, buffing, fanning... They are all designed to a) stop the crying and b) get the infant to relax physically.

It is not easy to fall asleep if you are crying. In fact, it's virtually impossible. Nor is it easy to fall asleep if your body is coiled like a spring. Relaxation, both mental and physical, is a prerequisite for sound sleep for every human being, big or small. It is also a prerequisite for falling back to sleep if you have woken up during the night, which we all do from time to time (even if we don't actually remember).

The opposite of peace is anxiety.

An infant's default condition, so to speak, is survival anxiety. All infants, by being driven out of the womb when nourishment and oxygen are cut off, are born out of the jaws of death with survival anxiety in their baggage. This survival anxiety must be allayed immediately and continuously.

All people know instinctively that what crying infants need, first and foremost, is food. It is only when their stomachs are full that other kinds of well-being are possible. That goes for us grown-ups too.

You can never give a newborn too much food. It will come out one end or the other.

A full stomach allays survival anxiety to a large extent, but it doesn't eradicate it. However full their little tummies are, infants are still helpless and vulnerable, utterly incapable of surviving on their own. If they fall to the ground, they can't even get up. If they don't starve, they can still freeze to death, and being devoured by wild animals is always a possibility.

All infants are instinctively aware of this from the moment they are born. All infants become nervous when handled tentatively or overcautiously. Firm, decisive handling is what is needed to make them feel secure. Although, obviously, they have never fallen, they are mortally afraid – quite literally – of falling to what they think is the ground, where they will quickly meet their doom.

There is nothing equivocal about the strategies in the *Good-Night's-Sleep Cure*. When you apply them, you will not be caressing your child's head, stomach or back. You will not be tenderly stroking that little cheek or picking her up to carry her around dejectedly in your anxious embrace. You will handle your child very firmly. You will be able to *calm* your child instead of alarming her even more, and you will be astonished over how effective these strategies are.

Now you will understand why.

This sense of calm must be brought about *immediately*. As a result, you cannot expect to get any sleep yourself during the first two nights of the *Good-Night's-Sleep Cure*. You must be unwaveringly prepared to intervene *instantly*.

During the third and fourth nights, you will be able to doze now and then, sometimes for several hours at a time, but you will have to stay alert enough to swing into action at a moment's notice.

As you will see in the Tool Box section and as you have seen in the parental reports I have cited, this so-called jingle has an enormous, almost magical, significance. It consists of a rhythmic goodnight jingle that is repeated four times in a row – a somewhat more sophisticated version of 'Happy Birthday' if you like. It is with this jingle that you will round off and finish all your physical interventions during this cure.

During the second night, the jingle will take on increasing significance, which means that when your child wakes up, you will try the jingle first rather than rushing into the child's room immediately. When you hear that the situation warrants it, you will be giving your child the opportunity to fall back to sleep herself without your having to intervene physically.

As early as the second night, you will probably hear how your child 'answers' your jingle and needs no more reassurance. You will then have made a contact with your child that is completely new to you. Communication is happening – a dialogue! You will experience a feeling that is as well-documented as it is euphoric. And that is just the treatment for a wounded parental heart.

If there is a pacifier in the picture, you will dispense with it the first night so that genuine mutual communication is possible. Your infant will forget all about the pacifier in a single night.

Calming an infant is not difficult. The strategies in the *Good-Night's-Sleep Cure* are so effective that you will be astonished at how easy it is. (The exception is the first time, when your child will quite naturally wonder what on earth is going on and whether you really know what you are doing. It can take anything from 20 to 45 minutes to give your answer reassuringly enough – but this will only happen once.)

If you are to be able to calm an infant who is upset for whatever reason, your own composure must be rock solid.

And that has not been the case thus far, or you would not be holding this book in your hand.

Human beings have been imbued with a powerful protective instinct that doesn't just extend to their own offspring. An infant's cries affect everyone. Not even a pin-stripe-clad childless male, intent on clawing his way up the career ladder, who spends his life rushing from one ultra-important meeting to another, briefcase in hand, remains unaffected by a crying baby. And he reacts with anxiety. He might not stop – he doesn't have the time – but he casts worried glances around him. *Where's the mother? Why doesn't someone do something? Is that kid all alone in the world?*

An infant's cries immediately awaken our instinct to protect life. We all know, just as a newborn baby does, that it is game over for human infants who fall to the ground, be it literally or metaphorically. The wolf will take them. Infants cry in their survival anxiety, and the instinct to survive is the strongest instinct we have. Without it, the human species would have died out long ago. Instead, we have conquered the world, and we didn't do it by abandoning one another – especially not the young children who keep the species going.

A more or less latent fear for our skins is something we all have in common. Where young children are concerned, parental responsibility for their welfare goes hand in hand with the protective instinct, which is fuelled – naturally enough – by anxiety.

Consequently, living by the axiom cited above – *If you are to be able to calm an infant who is upset for whatever reason, your own composure must be rock solid* – is easier said than done.

If you have ever been fearful that the archetypal wolf might come for you, then you probably know what the antidote is: the common sense that you have acquired over the course of your life, self-knowledge, knowledge of the world, your own experience and that of others, and much more.

Conversations with family and friends can help allay your fears, but only if they don't add fuel to the fire. *No, you will never get yourself out of this. You may as well give up now because you don't have a chance!*

This is hardly what you need to hear.

What you want is their encouragement and their respect as your fellow human beings, even if they perhaps don't quite understand what is so awful about, well, your survival anxiety. You want their soothing perspective on things in the form of simple words, spoken with conviction: *Things are going to work out. You will get through this. You are not alone in the world. Everything will be fine. You CAN!*

This is what you need to hear. You can take these words to heart, provided that you feel that you are understood, truly understood, rather than steamrollered with hearty clichés or waved away with lofty indifference.

The friends you would definitely not talk to about your apparently insurmountable problems are those who are drowning in anxiety themselves. The blind aren't very good at leading the blind. You would confide in someone you trusted, someone you regarded as strong, sensible, experienced and knowledgeable.

And we are not talking solely about 'personal' problems here. If you encountered problems in your professional life, you would seek out someone who could conceivably help you. If you are staring bankruptcy in the face, it doesn't make much sense to seek advice from someone whose business has just been seized by the bank.

If you think about it, you will understand that your young child, whose survival anxiety you have not been able to allay thus far, must be allowed to experience your own unshakable composure in order to feel a sense of calm herself.

And you will understand why young children who cry hysterically calm down in the presence of some people but remain hysterical in the presence of others (usually anxious parents). You will understand how I – a complete stranger in a completely unfamiliar house in a completely unfamiliar room – have personally been able to help hundreds of children over the years. More often than not these children have been in throes of the so-called eight-month anxiety. I have been able to give them *peace*.

It wasn't more anguish you were after when you sought help. You didn't want to see your friends burst into tears over your deplorable situation. You weren't fishing for pity. You wanted their sympathy, yes, but you didn't want to pull them into the dumps with you. You wanted understanding and a hearing from someone who cared, but the last thing you wanted was mute despair. You were looking for help!

Survival anxiety is a messy blend of fear for your life, anguish over the struggle to survive, and a fear of going under, mentally, physically or both. If life and limb are to be secured, if a safe haven is to be had, if body and mind are to be stabilized in a more or less functional way, first and foremost you must regain your inner *peace*.

Infants don't have any peace to regain. Survival anxiety sinks its claws into them before they are even born. The child has to leave the familiar, peaceful existence of the womb weighed down with the conviction that *I will never be able to manage this by myself.* Once the lifeline is cut, complete helplessness becomes a fact of life.

Gripped by survival anxiety, the infant screams. And screams. And screams. The protective instincts of the parents immediately crank into high gear. It is life itself that is at stake, personified by this little baby.

It is not just anxiety that is awakened. *'Why doesn't anyone do something?'* asked the pin-strip suit as he hurried by. The protective instinct demands action.

The child needs food. Without food, we can't live. But food is not enough. A range of other measures must be taken to guarantee the child's life.

One 'measure' that God and Nature have ensured is up and running in advance is the preparedness of the parents to love this little baby, who has been born with the magic wand of love in her hand.

What must also be assured is *peace.* An infant has no peace to fall back on. It has to be put in place *now.*

Your own inner peace, which you have hopefully rediscovered with the help of common sense, knowledge and experience, friendship, prudence and the ability to put things in perspective didn't solve your problems. They remained. But you are now able to deal with them, which you weren't before.

As long as you were weighed down by your anguish, sleepless, and in mental agony, you didn't stand a chance. You found yourself in a vicious cycle, and things just kept getting worse. In the end, there was not a glimmer of hope on the horizon. There was absolutely nothing you could take any joy in, tortured as you were by survival anxiety.

Your baby is in the same boat. Young children are made of exactly the same stuff as we adults.

Restless nights, when you doze fitfully but never really fall into a sound sleep, are as burdensome to little people as they are for big ones.

You have no doubt been told the opposite:

- *'Young children take the sleep they need all by themselves'*. But you didn't when you lay tossing and turning, incapable of relaxing because of all the fears that were plaguing you! You *couldn't* take the sleep you needed. You desperately wanted to, but it just didn't happen.
- *'Young children don't need that much sleep.'* Why not? You do. All the sleep you can get. You're exhausted. Why wouldn't your infant be? Look at her pale skin, the dark circles under her eyes, the weary, blank stares devoid of even the faintest sparkle.
- *'All young children wake up during the night for their first few years'*. It's because of this, that or the other, you have been told, and it's completely normal, not to say inevitable. *'Sleep? Forget it!'* Constant waking for the first two or three years comes with the territory so get over it. But how is it that, thanks to the *Good-Night's-Sleep Cure,* young children – even as young as four months – are being able to sleep soundly and continuously for twelve hours per night, instead of waking up all the time?

And the worst of it is that you simply can't cope. There comes a time when the status quo has to be rejected. There comes a time to doubt the facts you have been fed.

When did someone decide that young children are incapable of sleeping through the night? Are they really incapable of sleeping? Didn't you sleep when you were young? You are fast-tracked to divorce court and tearing your hair out. Don't all these explanations start to sound a little contrived?

There you stand with my book in your hand, on which you are pinning your last hope. *We have tried everything.*

And now you're suffering from more than the sleep deprivation that threatens your marriage, your work, your sex life and all the other joys that life brings. You are also feeling like a complete failure as a parent. The sleep problem has overwhelmed you. Hearing how normal it all is – *this just goes with the territory when you have kids* – isn't much help. You are not in any shape to cope anymore, no matter how much you think you should be.

Is that really all there is to life when you have kids? *Coping?*

Problems are there to be solved. You feel you weren't up to the task. Human beings want to solve problems, not succumb to them.

Everyone, including you, knows that young children are helpless. They are completely dependent on the care and attention of the adult world. And they want to do more than just survive; they want to *live*.

Living means feeling – and expressing – joy, satisfaction and contentment over a life well lived. With all your love, you parents should be good enough to succeed in achieving and confirming that joy and contentment! Everyone expects it of you. Even more important, you expect it of yourselves. But every prolonged scream, which seems to last forever, indicates the opposite: you are failures as parents. *It doesn't matter what I do. I feel like the world's worst mother.*

This is torture every bit as cruel as sleep deprivation. Feeling that you are a terrible parent is the same as feeling you are a terrible human being. If you can't look after your child sufficiently well to give her peace and contentment, in spite of the fact you have all the prerequisites at your disposal, both emotionally and materially, you aren't really much to write home about. Having children, being a parent should be the most natural thing in the world! People have been having kids since the year dot and they obviously were able to look after them properly or none of us would be here. *One* newborn hardly turned the world upside down for a family that maybe had eleven other kids that had to be fed and eighteen cows that had to be milked.

How did they do it? How does anybody do it? *Why can't I do it?*

Your self-confidence has crumbled and that's bad enough. But you have been drained of self-esteem too. It's trickled down into a chasm of powerlessness along with the bitter tears you have shed. That's even worse. Once our self-esteem is undermined, we are on the edge of mental breakdown.

And it doesn't seem to matter how much you love this little child. It doesn't seem to matter how much you carry her around and comfort her or how often you bring her into your bed. It doesn't seem to matter how often you give her the pacifier, or yourself if you are breastfeeding. You think you are going mad. You wish your child had better parents and you wish you had never been born.

Here I beg leave to indulge in a polemical digression. It is no surprise that birth rates are falling in rich countries and that these countries desperately want them to rise. Taking joy in young children has fallen by the wayside. It has become unbearably complicated to have kids.

Day and night parents are expected to satisfy their child's insatiable demands for physical and emotional closeness – which hardly leaves any wiggle room for another child. Since we are expected to work outside the home at our earliest opportunity and become independent, self-fulfilled and economically self-sufficient women (and men), we have to drag our perpetually guilty consciences to work with us because we feel we are depriving our children of their need for intimacy for days on end. Thus, we feel compelled to compensate for this repeated neglect with nocturnal company, evening entertainment and frenetic weekend stimulation. (And things of course. The average Swedish pre-schooler has 536 toys. And a Lego set with a million pieces counts as *one*.)

This same society, which never tires of emphasizing the importance of family and makes a religion out of the idea of intimacy and companionship between parent and child, through its actions makes it all but impossible for parents to live and function with their children in a family worthy of the name. The experts, who are so quick to point the finger of moral opprobrium at parents and who place *separation anxiety* on a par with the Seven Deadly Sins, grovel enthusiastically before the idol of corporate profit and joyfully advocate warehousing children virtually anywhere, just as long as it is not in the tender embrace of their mothers and fathers.

The logical contortions are legion. We are all great parents. No one knows our children better than we do. We are the foremost and only experts; yet, in the next breath, it is asserted that it is in the home at the hands of the parents that the most appalling abuse occurs; the home is a toxic miasma of assault, drug abuse and violence. If children fare badly, they fare worst with those who love them best. Parents are the best and the worst, authorities and punching bags, white as snow and black as sin all at the same time.

Stress and anxiety are the daily bread that ought to consist of wholesome ingredients, baked without sugar of course. Sleep deprivation is to be endured but parents are to be well rested anyway. Mothers are to be free, self-sufficient, independent, and politically correct, *and* live in a state of extended womb symbiosis with their children. Fathers are to shoulder their recently conferred responsibilities, parental and domestic, clean the house, do the dishes, prepare the meals, change the diapers, play with and comfort their children, generally relieve the pressure on their wives *and* work full-time.

Divorce and the dissolution of the home are traumatic events for children, yet divorce is regarded as relatively trivial – in Sweden, 40% of parents drift apart before their children turn one, 50% before they turn two – just as long as the children are allowed to bounce back and forth between their parents and are loved by both equally. There is of course an inconvenient proviso that forbids parents from loving any children that come along with their new partners *too* much because the children from marriage number one, who were first in line, might feel marginalized – because they *are* marginalized. The paradoxes are mind-boggling! I could go on forever, but that would not be in keeping with a chapter entitled *Peace*. (Or would it?)

Let me now conclude: when people stop bringing children into the society in which they live because they have come to understand that work and family are, practically and economically, mutually exclusive, they are giving that society a failing grade. They are saying that they don't think that such a society has a future. And that is a death sentence because children are the future.

Back to peace! Remember the safari?

If you read the safari allegory and succeeded in imagining that you were the one making the journey, you will remember that it didn't take much to enable you to feel at peace when you embarked on the great adventure. Your positive expectations knew no bounds.

As for the guide, who put a team together to lead the safari, you had nothing but confidence in him. You thought he was *fabulous. A soul on fire, knowledgeable and confident.*

It is precisely this kind of simple, positive peace that you will be able to give your child – at long last!

The spontaneous trust you felt is comparable to the instinctive trust newborns feel for their parents. This trust is innate and wreathed in positive expectations. The child you have in your care assumes that you and your assistant(s) will take care of her in the best possible way. Otherwise, it wouldn't be much of a life! In similar fashion, you and your nature-loving sojourners counted on the guide and his assistants to take care of you in the best possible way. Otherwise, it wouldn't be much of a safari.

What was it you experienced? You felt you were *adequately and professionally looked after.* The result was peace of mind.

How much did the guide have to exert himself to achieve that? Not much. Your trust in him was there already, just as an infant's instinctive trust is. You were handed over to him, and you wouldn't have been able to manage without him, but you didn't distrust him. Quite the contrary, you were prepared to both admire and learn from him. He didn't need to *earn* your trust. It was enough that he was chosen to be your guide. You assumed that he knew what he was doing.

Kids assume that too.

On the other hand, the guide could of course *forfeit* the trust you so willingly gave him. You remember his little performance in the tent. There you were on your bunk with chattering teeth and a pounding heart, while a pride of lions was roaring outside the tent. He left his gun at the entrance and, to your astonishment, came over to you, tilted his head to one side and looked *worried.* He felt sorry for you because you were so frightened. He suggested that you and he could cuddle a little, dance, have a 'cakey-wakey'.

60

In the end, you were ticked off at him. What you wanted was *peace of mind*, and that was not to be had from him, standing there and wallowing in his own worries as he was. You thought that he should darn well be standing outside the tent, his gun cocked, doing what he was hired for. He should be keeping the lions away!

Only when that base was covered, would you have been able to sleep soundly and gather your strength for bird watching the next morning.

Your trust in him was a little frayed around the edges, but he hadn't quite forfeited it yet. We all have our bad days. You decided to regard his sudden lack of confidence and his disconcerting anxiety attack as a one-off psychotic break.

The protective instinct is awakened in all of us when infants cry. The raison d'être of this instinct is, or at least should be, the bestowal of *peace of mind*. We should not be aggravating an infant's survival anxiety by becoming anxious ourselves.

This sense of peace is what young children need more than anything else. But I would bet that when you sought explanations for why your baby kept waking up and screaming all night long and wondered desperately what on earth you were supposed to do, neither the experts nor the people around told you that *your child needs peace of mind.*

Instead, you were told to look for problems. Something must be wrong because your baby isn't sleeping. Colic? Gas? Stomach ache? Physical illness has to be ruled out first, so it's off to the doctor. Allergies perhaps? Speculations run wild. Teething? Nightmares? Fear of the dark? A genetic defect? Is the baby too warm, too cold, too wet, too dry? Is the baby being deprived of physical or emotional intimacy? Should the baby be stuck to the mother's breast 24/7? *We have tried everything!*

Your baby doesn't benefit from a frantic search for possible medical problems or ever more desperate attempts to comfort, anymore than you would benefit from the guide feeling sorry for you and getting uptight himself. It is *peace of mind* your baby needs.

The *Good-Night's-Sleep Cure* gives you the calming strategies you need, all of which stem from your own unshakable composure. *An attitude that says that everything you do is so obviously right it ought to be self-evident* is one of them.

To reiterate: you will be astonished at how easy it is to give an anxious infant peace of mind. Your little one, who is plagued by survival anxiety, is no exception.

Children need and want peace of mind.

Just like we do.

2. SECURITY

All young children must be calmed if they are to relax, fall silent and then fall asleep.

And, if and when you decide to embark upon the *Good-Night's-Sleep Cure*, you will see that it is not that hard to calm even a hysterically crying infant once you know what to do.

When you manage that, your self-esteem will make a comeback!

At this point, you may be tempted to close the book and put it away because you figure you've cracked the code. Now you know the drill. *Don't* pick the baby up. Calm her where she is lying. Look how good I am at it, you say to yourself.

And indeed you are. But at the risk of sounding like a killjoy, you mustn't stop there. You must take the next step. In addition to peace of mind, you must provide *a sense of security*.

Your baby will be content with nothing less.

And this is perfectly understandable if you cast your mind back to your first night on safari, when you ate a good dinner, had yourself a nightcap as the sun went down and then retired to your private tent as content as you could be. You were well fed, relaxed and full of joyous expectations for the next day.

But then you heard a lion roar uncomfortably close to the tent, and you naturally had to ask yourself what the *security* situation was out there in the bush.

Did you dare sleep soundly? Could you really believe that life and limb were not at risk? The tent was made of material so flimsy that any predator could rip it to shreds as easily as you could tear a piece of paper in half.

'Is the wolf coming to get me now?' is precisely the question that an infant asks.

So even if that little tummy is full – and it must be, more than full hopefully – your child is still to be lulled into a sense of absolute security. Peace of mind for the moment is not enough.

So, you must not content yourself with the wonderful breakthrough that you achieved during the first two nights when, with the help of the prescribed strategies, you succeeded in giving your child *peace of mind* so that she could sleep. If you stop there and think you are out of the woods because you can now buff your baby into silence or rock her into tranquillity, *insecurity* will set in during nights three and four.

Your baby will allow herself to be calmed, as long as you apply the appropriate strategies, but she will not wake up less frequently but more – again. Whereupon you will buff, rock, fan and jingle for all you are worth... And before you know what hit you, you will find yourself standing beside your child's bed for half the night (or all night) – again.

Your baby has nothing against the way you are handling her, she just protests as soon as you stop. She isn't sleeping through the night at all!

So why isn't it working you ask yourself. Everything was going so well. *What did I do wrong?*

Insecurity has sunk its claws into you – again. That's why it's not working. Insecurity is the opposite of security.

Once you have understood the fundamental importance of a sense of security and learned to communicate this in a way that convinces your child, the *Good-Night's-Sleep Cure can't* fail.

'But why wouldn't my child feel *secure?*' I hear you cry a little distrustfully. You and your partner have taken every conceivable precaution to protect the little life that has been placed in your care and for which you are responsible!

You both make sure that your baby is never exposed to danger. You never leave her alone. You always look both ways when you cross the street with the baby carriage. You have laid out a small fortune to ensure your child's safety. You take no risks. You do everything humanly possible to protect yourselves – and above all your child – from the wolf in all its guises day and night, home and away, indoors and outdoors.

And you succeed. *You* know that your child is safe and so does your partner.

But your child doesn't.

If your infant thought she was safe, you wouldn't be holding this book in your hand. Your child would be sleeping at night because *sleeping at night comes naturally to human beings.* It is as natural as it is necessary.

When God in his wisdom divided day from night, both men and beasts gratefully took their repose in the darkness. Such was the theory and such is the practice.

And children are made of the same stuff as we adults.

Young children who feel *secure*, who know that they are protected from the wolf in all its guises, do not wake up time after time during the night, regardless of whether they sleep on their backs or their stomachs, in their own beds and rooms or with their parents, on their mothers' breasts or standing on their heads in the closet. They sleep. And they sleep well.

And they will happily sleep twelve hours a night from the age of four months.

On the other hand, young children who do *not* feel secure, who have *not* allowed themselves to be convinced that they are protected from the wolf in all its guises, will continue to wake up. They will wake up time after time, day and night, after periods of sleep that are not only brief but also fitful.

Time after time, they are gripped by survival anxiety. Time after time, they ask the same anguished question: *Is the wolf coming to get me?*

Your task, should you decide to embark upon the *Good-Night's-Sleep Cure*, is to answer this question *in a way that satisfies your child.*

Human beings are fragile creatures. If we were cast out in the dead of winter, we wouldn't last one night. We don't have claws, fangs or pelts. We can't run very fast if we have to escape danger. Our muscular strength is so unimpressive that we need weapons to fight our enemies and defend our lives. We are easy marks for all kinds of 'wolves'. We are prone to illness, we can't take much stress and we can't survive alone.

This frail creation called *homo sapiens* has subjugated the planet.

No wonder that the first order of business for the human race was to ensure its physical *security*, since the wolf in all its guises was waiting at every turn, poised to wipe humanity off the face of the earth!

And along comes your infant, the product of millions of years of evolution, who knows in her bone marrow that she would not stand a chance of even getting a meal all by herself. The wolf that is called survival anxiety began to snap at her heels in the womb, as soon as the food and oxygen supply was cut off. The child was forced out – there was no alternative if she was to survive – only to be confronted on her arrival in this world by the very wolf she was fleeing from.

You know your house is Fort Knox. In a world at peace, a world where material resources are virtually limitless, you know that you can give your child a comfortable, secure life and that there is nothing to be afraid of.

Even so, every hour of every day, you take a whole raft of *preventive measures* designed to keep the wolf at bay.

You look both ways when you cross the street. You are meticulous about paying bills so the bank doesn't repossess your house. You eat a healthy diet to minimize the risk of illness or death.

You are especially careful at night, when you know you are vulnerable because you are asleep. You bolt the front door. You make sure the windows are secure so no thieves or murderers can get in. You activate the burglar alarm if you have one. You might even have gotten yourself a guard dog to warn you about any unexpected visitors. You blow out the candles, and check the stove and all appliances. You cast a glance at the smoke alarm, looking for that reassuring blink. You give the whole house or apartment a quick tour before you go to bed to make sure that everything is as it should be.

And then you look in on your child – one last time.

Humans first built shelters to protect themselves from wild animals. The safer the shelters, the more secure they felt when they gave themselves over to life sustaining sleep.

If they didn't feel *secure* and protected from the wolf – in war, at sea or on safari in the bush – they either had to stand guard themselves or get someone to do it for them.

Today surveillance methods have moved far beyond individuals literally standing guard, but it wasn't that long ago that soldiers walked the perimeter of their camp, ships had a look-out in the crow's nest, and people on safari had guards posted outside their tents, which was the scenario we placed you in.

Soldiers in the field took turns doing guard duty while their comrades slept. Keen eyed and alert, they would keep watch on enemy lines in the darkness until they were relieved and could sleep themselves. If there was the slightest indication that the enemy was on the move, the commander would be informed and the unit readied for battle.

Their task was not to tiptoe around their comrades to make sure they had fallen asleep comfortably after counting lice. Had they done so, their sleeping comrades would probably have scrambled to their feet terrified. Was the enemy moving? Had the perimeter been breached?

The lookout in the crow's nest kept watch for icebergs, enemy ships, vessels that had strayed off course and anything else that spelled danger. He also had a duty to immediately report anything suspicious to the captain and the crew.

His task was not to sit in the captain's cabin and hold his hand, and if he had bothered his crew mates while they were sleeping, they probably would have made him walk the plank.

The task of your guide/guard on the safari was to ensure that you got a good sleep, which you desperately wanted because you had to be up early the next morning to go bird watching. He stood guard outside the tent. He didn't bother you with his fears, anxieties and insecurities. He didn't burden you with his own need for cosy nocturnal company. (Except when he suffered that temporary psychotic break of course, a transgression for which you magnanimously forgave him on the understanding that it would not reoccur.) He and his assistants guarded the entire party so that all of you could sleep soundly in your tents – and fall back to sleep if you were woken up by roaring lions.

The guard respected your need for sleep. *Secure* sleep.

'No lion would dare approach the camp,' he reassured you when, with a pounding heart, you discreetly hailed him to make sure he was still there. 'And if one were stupid enough to try, he would only do it once. No worries there.'

That is precisely the message that you will convey to your infant.

'You can rest easy. We are watching over you. We know the danger and we will hold it at bay. Your survival is guaranteed.'

I will say it again. Once you understand the fundamental importance of a sense of security and you learn to convey this sense of total security in a way that convinces *your child*, the *Good-Night's-Sleep Cure* can't fail.

But first, let us take a long hard look at the things that will virtually guarantee failure!

I want to give you the heads-up about these particular wolves that are lurking in the bushes so you can avoid them. They are:

- Revealing your own insecurity to your child.
- Letting your child lead you instead of assuming a leadership role yourself.
- Operating in permanent crisis mode.

The Art of Failure 1: Revealing your own insecurity to your child
It's an easy mistake to make. You *are* insecure. It's just the way things are.

If you were an experienced child-minder of the old school or you had had eight children before, you wouldn't be tearing your hair out. You certainly wouldn't be tearing your hair out in front of your child. You would instinctively know how to cope with any problems that came up.

Because come up they do. And you aren't an experienced child-minder of the old school. Everything that happens – if and when you decide to embark upon the *Good-Night's-Sleep Cure* – is a first for both you and your child.

The *Good-Night's-Sleep Cure* is a process. It breaks new ground, rather than just following the old familiar rut. This is not a static method. The simple calming technique that you are beginning with is not enough to achieve the result you want: *enjoyment!*

The first two or three nights of the *Good-Night's-Sleep Cure* usually go off without a hitch, even though the first night, when the old patterns are broken with the attendant, sometimes violent, protests from the child, requires its share of intensive, single-minded work.

When peace descends, which usually *starts* to happen during the second night, when the so-called jingle assumes more and more significance (soon to take over completely), the child poses new questions. And displays new reactions. To your amazement, you begin to hear something that can't really be described as anything else but a form of angry swearing.

You will start to hear cries that are entirely new to you. What do they mean? How are you to answer them?

She is unhappy! He is in distress! *I must comfort!*

And in you go to give this comfort, just as you have learned to do and that has worked so well, in spite of the fact that the jingle was supposed to take over by now.

You are not calming your child in the sense of convincing her that everything is as it should be. You are calming in order to *comfort.*

This of course is perfectly understandable. Unfortunately, however, *comfort is of no use to a child who is seeking security.*

It is of no more use than the 'comfort' your guide gave you when he experienced his temporary psychotic break in the tent, put down his gun, and approached your cot brimming with empathy.

'Oh dear! Are you scared? I feel so sorry for you!' He tilted his head to one side and said, 'I can lie down beside you for a while and stroke you if you like.'

Stroke you? You were so petrified, you didn't know which end was up. It was very kind of him, but... the lions were roaring just outside the tent! Three of them! Their roars were so ear-splitting, they might just as well have been inside the tent with you. How could he believe that they would disappear if he lay down beside you and stroked you?

You were frightened as you lay there listening to those lions (real or imaginary). But comfort wasn't what you needed. You weren't unhappy or depressed. It was perhaps sad that you were so frightened your teeth were chattering, but the cure for fear is not empathy. It's *security*.

It is this *Attitude of Self-Evidence* – one of the most important strategies in the *Good-Night's-Sleep Cure* – that better than anything imbues your child with a sense of absolute security.

The Art of Failure 2: Letting your child lead you instead of assuming a leadership role yourself

This is a tough one these days. New parents are bombarded with the message that it is the child who should decide.

But young children cannot decide anything. They haven't the foggiest notion of the rules that govern a place that they have never been to before.

After all, you didn't when you were on safari.

How are meals provided for example? Out in the bush, restaurants are few and far between. Does everyone just cook food over an open fire? What time is dinner? What about breakfast and lunch?

It's not that you were worried. You just wanted to know. You and your fellow sojourners were asking yourselves how exactly this safari was *organized*.

The guide assembled you and his assistants at the airport. He walked you through every last detail, including food preparation. There would be a mobile kitchen and here was the cook. (Appreciative applause.) Every day, the expedition would stop for supplies and you would have an opportunity to stock up on personal items. All your needs would be satisfied so everyone can relax. (Delighted laughter.)

You trusted the safari guide immediately. It was obvious that he was an old hand at all this. From the very first day, you felt *adequately and professionally looked after.*

You certainly didn't sign up for this safari to hunt your own food, or to lie sleepless all night with a pounding heart. You wanted to devote yourself one hundred percent to enjoying the fantastic adventure that awaited you.

This is exactly how infants feel.

Let's say the guide, when he meets you at the airport with his assistants, does not present an organized itinerary. He provides you with no information about meals or anything else.

Instead he says, 'Sorry guys, but I actually have no idea about any of this stuff. We'll just have to play it by ear. You're the ones that decided to go on this junket, so you are going to have to decide how we are going to organize everything. *I* don't know. I've actually never been on a safari before.'

How would you have reacted?

You and your fellow sojourners would have probably looked at each other in utter bewilderment and wondered what on earth was going on. Didn't the guide know what he was doing? Wasn't he the man in charge? Were *you* supposed to organize the safari?

Your spontaneous reaction would have been insecurity.

Insecurity is the opposite of security.

Infants are creatures of habit.

It is very easy to introduce routines for a young child. And it's popular too.

Even at two months, infants gratefully accept – and, I would argue, expect – all that confident leadership, fixed times and established routines involve.

You are a creature of habit yourself. It's hardly surprising since most of us mortals are. I wouldn't mind betting that you are dependent on a hearty breakfast and two cups of coffee in the morning, lunch at one, a coffee break in the afternoon and dinner between seven and eight at night.

But what are you really doing when you eat dinner if I may ask? Are you really eating simply to stay alive? Or do you indulge yourself in an appetizer and dessert, as well as a main course perhaps accompanied by a glass of good wine? Do you really need all that?

Of course not, you retort. You could survive on 800 calories a day!

And no doubt you could. All those extra goodies that you eat and drink, which are not at all essential for survival, you partake of because *they produce a sense of well-being.*

You *enjoy* food and drink. You don't think it is a chore to eat. Eating hardly makes you an object of pity.

You also enjoy a good night's sleep, that long lost friend with whom you will hopefully be reacquainted before too much longer. You don't think sleeping is a chore. The fact that you need your sleep doesn't make you an object of pity either.

The same holds true for young children.

Established routines generate not only energy but also *pleasure.*

You didn't go on safari because you wanted to hunt for survival or take charge of organizing the whole enterprise. You went on safari because you wanted to devote yourself one hundred percent to enjoying the fantastic adventure that awaited you.

That is exactly what an infant wants.

Young children should be enjoyed and enjoy themselves!

When you assume your role as leader, instead of handing it over to your child, you give your child the same sense of security that you experienced at the airport when you realized that your guide had every angle covered. You immediately understood that the guide and his assistants knew their business.

Even if you weren't directly worried about anything, you still felt relief. Your needs were going to be catered to right down to your morning coffee!

This first safari was *terra incognita* for you. Even if you were only planning to take pictures rather than actually hunt (let's say), you would still be in close proximity to wild animals out there on the savannah. You would be spending your nights in a tent, alone and unarmed. There is no way you would have been able to cater to your own needs whether it was getting your morning coffee or escaping from a blood-thirsty lion. You and your fellow sojourners would have had to place yourselves entirely in the hands of the *guide*.

That is what infants have to do.

Infants can't cater to their needs anymore than you and your fellow sojourners would have been able to on this first safari of their lives. They expect the guide and his assistants to take responsibility for their well-being and security.

And they have every right to. What choice do they have? Like you on your safari, they want to survive. They want their survival anxiety allayed, and they want to *enjoy life*.

The latter is impossible until the former is assured.

If and when you decide to embark upon the *Good-Night's-Sleep Cure*, fixed times and routines are the first item of business. You will draw up a schedule based on your infant's needs.

This schedule, which you will meticulously follow (with a maximum margin of error of fifteen minutes), means that you will continuously be taking *preventive measures* to keep the wolf at bay, just as you do to secure your own existence.

You will always be one step ahead.

You have understood that your child's needs out here in the world aren't that much different from your own, and now you can meet them preventively. You are no longer patching and filling after the damage has been done in a more or less fruitless attempt to make your child happy.

By establishing a schedule, you are assuming your leadership role. You become the *guide* that your child expects you to be.

The idea that your child would have the desire or the capability to decide how the days and nights should be organized on her first terrestrial expedition is, as you now understand, absurd. Just as the idea of your organizing a safari is absurd. If you and your fellow sojourners were faced with the prospect of leading the safari yourselves because the guide and his assistants were clueless, you would immediately feel *insecure*.

By introducing fixed times and routines that enable you to meet your child's needs continuously and preventively, you are assuming a leadership role and in so doing you are bestowing a sense of *security*. You are giving your child a framework within which she can rest secure, enjoy life and avoid having to worry about how she would guard her interests out there in the world – which by definition would be impossible anyway.

At this point, you may sigh. Schedules sound so dull! Are they really necessary? Won't every day feel like a straightjacket? Can we even go out the front door if we have to keep to a schedule that literally only gives us fifteen minutes worth of wiggle room?

You're right. You won't be straying far from home during the cure itself, when *peace of mind* is established.

Ditto for the follow-up week, when a *sense of security* is being established.

Peace of mind and a sense of security require, well, peace and security, and convincing your child that a regime change has in fact taken place is best done *at home*. Just ponder your own associations with your home, your refuge from the world!

But later?

Once you have conscientiously worked your way through the *Good-Night's-Sleep Cure* and let it settle for a week or two, you will have an infant who can be fed by anyone, put to bed by anyone and who can sleep anywhere. And stay cheerful through it all!

As long as you *stick to the schedule*.

As you will see, the routines you have introduced are not dependent on people or places. They are only dependent on time.

You will have to take preventive measures if you travel to the other side of the world with your child to make up for the change in time zone, but you will have a happy little companion on safari with you. That I can promise you!

When your infant knows that she is *secure*, her capacity to *enjoy life* will soon be in full bloom. Then you will have the most amiable, the happiest, and the most flexible traveling companion you could wish for wherever your feet decide to take you!

The Art of Failure 3: Operating in permanent crisis mode

One summer, when I was eight years old, I visited my Aunt Elinda. She lived by herself in a log cabin out in the country.

One afternoon clouds started to gather. Thunder rumbled. By evening the sky was criss-crossed by forks of lightning. The house had no lightning rod, so Aunt Elinda was vigilant.

'Before you go to bed, pack a bag,' she told me. 'And put out your traveling clothes. Don't forget your overcoat. Sleep in your underwear, not your nightie.'

We would have to leave the house in a hurry if it was struck by lightning, she explained. I didn't really want to go to bed that night.

And sure enough, Aunt Elinda woke me up in the middle of the night. 'Get ready! I'll wait in the hall. Hurry!'

I jumped out of bed and struggled into my clothes, grabbed my suitcase and jacket and ran out into the hall. There was Aunt Elinda sitting on the floor in her hat and coat staring morosely out the window. She was listening and counting. 'One, two, three... it's getting closer! The next lightening bolt is going to hit us!'

There we sat with our suitcases, ready to flee, and counted the seconds between the thunder and the lightning. The shorter the interval, the closer the lightning. The closer the lightning, the greater the danger.

Crisis!

If lightning struck the log cabin and set it ablaze, we would have to run for our lives, so the front door was unlocked. Emergency supplies of food and clothing and rain gear were all packed. Aunt Elinda was in disaster relief mode and she had thought of everything.

When she finally deemed the danger to be over, I was allowed to go back to bed.

'But don't unpack!' she called after me. 'Lightning really can strike twice in the same place!'

Dazed, I crept back to bed. I had never been exposed to Nature's wrath before. There was a lot to be afraid of. The house could go up in flames at any moment. If I happened to be asleep, I'd go up in flames with it. There's no way I'd be able to get out in time. I would probably wake up when my clothes actually caught fire, but then it would be too late... It was a horrible thought, and it scared the living daylights out of the little girl I was back then. All eight-year-olds have more imagination than is good for them. I could see the flames licking my hands and feet, racing up my arms and legs, my hair exploding in a crown of fire, while the bed, the room, the whole house became an inferno... And then I died!

But none of that would happen. I would not burn to death. Aunt Elinda knew how to handle this *crisis*. When the proverbial wolf attacked with thunder and lightning and threatened to consume the house, Aunt Elinda went into emergency response mode for both of us.

She didn't deny the danger. She didn't say, 'Thunder is nothing to worry about!'

She recognized the danger. It was clear and present. The wolf was at the door.

And she didn't comfort me when I was afraid. She didn't say, 'Poor love, you're scared of thunder. I feel so sorry for you.'

Comfort isn't much use to someone who is seeking security.

Instead, she took sensible preventive measures that she deemed necessary to ensure our *security*.

When the storm blew over, she let me go back to bed. She didn't follow me into my bedroom. She didn't keep me awake. She didn't disturb me. She didn't make me anxious unless there was a real *crisis*.

Do you remember the story of the boy who cried wolf? 'Wolf! Wolf!' he shouted. The village declared a state of emergency. But the wolf never showed.

Again the boy cried, 'Wolf! Wolf!'

Again a state of emergency was declared. Primed and ready for anything, the villagers rallied to confront the threat. But yet again, the wolf didn't show.

The boy continued to shout. 'Wolf! Wolf!'

But now the villagers began to doubt the boy. The wolf never came. The boy was making it all up the villagers told each other. He probably thought it was amusing to watch the whole village go into emergency mode. He made things happen, which in turn made him feel important.

So the villagers decided they weren't going to let the boy make fools of them any longer. They just wanted to plod through their daily lives as usual and sleep well at night.

The day came, however, when the wolf really did come, and he had more than enough time to raise hell, since the boy's warning cries went unheeded. But that's another story.

In Gulliver's time, if we continue browsing through literature, a night watchman would wander the cobbled streets with a lantern shouting, '*All is well! All is well!*' at regular intervals.

All was well in the town, and its citizens could rest easy. That was the message.

And the citizens in the town want nothing more, the villagers in the fairy tale want nothing more, you on your safari out there in the bush want nothing more, and infants want nothing more than to rest easy.

God in his wisdom divided day from night, and both men and beasts gratefully took their repose in the darkness. Such was the theory and such is the practice. *Sleeping at night comes naturally to human beings.*

And kids are made of the same stuff as we grown-ups.

So why doesn't your child sleep? Why are you holding my book in your hand and desperately seeking the help that hitherto you haven't been able to find?

(Or haven't wanted to find? The Controlled Crying Method doesn't appeal to you I hope. Your child doesn't have to scream herself into an exhausted, resigned sleep, which is as fitful as your child is anxious. Nor should your child be subjected to the violent assault that drugging her with neuroleptics involves.)

Time after time, day and night, your child wakes up after sleep periods that are far too short and far too fitful. *We have tried everything.*

Now the situation has become unbearable. Your whole family is going under.

And now you suspiciously pose a question. If sleep at night comes naturally to people, even very little ones, how come *my* child can't sleep?

The answer is that you and your partner, with the best will in the world, have inadvertently declared a state of emergency.

You are operating in permanent crisis mode.

How did that happen?

Your infant has raised the warning flag, as infants do. *Help. Danger threatens.* And you have ridden to the rescue.

As we have seen, not even the most hardened pin-striped corporate climber can remain unmoved by an infant's cries. *Where's the mother? Why doesn't someone do something?*

That protective instinct that we all have is awakened. Even young children feel protective towards children who are even younger and more helpless than they are.

So you pick up your baby, who is crying out in her hour of need, and start looking for root causes.

You have taken every conceivable precaution. You have fed her, changed her, carried her, comforted her, taken her temperature, checked for teething problems, perhaps given her Panadol, taken her for a drive, carried her up and down the stairs, jumped and danced, cooed and stroked, massaged and caressed.

When one of you finally gets her to fall asleep in your arms, you carefully put her to bed again. Once down, she only sleeps for a little while – or doesn't sleep at all but starts to cry again.

It's really not that strange. After all, there is a wolf in the bed!

What you are doing when you pick up screaming infants, instead of calming them wherever they happen to be lying, is *saving* them. Through your actions you are saying:

'There's no way you can lie here! It's suicide! The wolf can take you whenever he likes! We have to get you somewhere safe!'

Every time you *save* an infant by protecting her with your body, you are confirming that she is in danger.

And that doesn't calm your child. Quite the contrary, you exacerbate her survival anxiety.

Your rescue effort calms her temporarily because you are providing physical protection with you body. Your body acts as a kind of air raid shelter. *The bombs are dropping! The wolf is coming!*

In the meantime, the wolf hops up on the bed from which you have just snatched your child. And there he waits with slavering jaws, set to pounce on his helpless prey.

So your child wakes up as soon as you put her down and promptly starts to cry. Survival anxiety sets in – yet again.

Your child's crying is born of this survival anxiety. *Is the wolf going to come for me?*

'Yes,' you answered. 'He is coming for you. Your life hangs by a thread. If I don't protect you with my body, you won't survive.'

Perhaps you have already been seduced into believing that your child's basic human need for emotional intimacy would be satisfied by nocturnal physical contact.

You think that the last thing physical contact conveys is the threat of *danger*.

For one thing, physical contact is not the same as emotional intimacy. That is a fact of life known only too well to everyone who has had bodily contact with another person without feeling love. The emotional intimacy on which we are all so dependent has to take place when we are *awake*. It is mutual, clear-eyed and warm. It's active.

For another, your physical presence during the night does not guarantee your child's *security*, just as the safari guide's did not when he put down his gun and offered to lie beside you, stroke you, comfort you and feel sorry for you. You told him to get out. You were indignant because you felt he should be doing his job. And that job was guaranteeing your nocturnal *security*.

You are doubling as an air raid shelter if and when let your child sleep beside you in your bed at night. The fact that you play this role as air raid shelter does not convey a sense of security to your child. Quite the contrary, it conveys a sense of *crisis*.

And that is why infants who are put down in the parental bed expect the parents to be there too. Always. They can't leave. They are and remain human shields against the wolf.

Your child's need for physical and emotional intimacy must be satisfied during the day! During the night, she has a basic human need for a sound, undisturbed, peaceful and secure sleep that must be tended to, a need that is just as essential if body and soul are to be kept together.

You child's sleep is hers and hers alone. It's sacred and must be given the reverence it deserves.

With the best will in the world, instead of conveying a sense of security and peace to your child, you have declared a state of *permanent emergency*.

'The war is coming! The wolf is coming!' You sound the alarm and confirm the danger as soon as the child asks the agonizing question: *Is the wolf coming for me?*

Through your anxious search for root causes, enthusiastically supported by those around you, you have actually invited the wolf in. *The wolf is probably coming!*

This situation you now find yourself in, as you desperately search for a solution to the sleep problem, has overwhelmed you. How much longer will you be able to stand it?

Not long I imagine. The dam will eventually burst.

Infants can't stand it for very long either.

No one can live in a permanent state of emergency.

During the Second World War, everyone knew there would be nightly air raids. When darkness fell, the air raid sirens wailed over the cities so that people would have time to seek safety in the shelters. And there they would wait until the all clear was sounded.

Today many countries are at war. If war hasn't actually been declared, a *state of emergency* has. Not everyone can take the sensible, preventive emergency measures that Aunt Elinda took when the storm clouds gathered.

How many nights in succession, and how many times per night, can people be pulled out of a sound sleep and seek shelter from falling bombs before they fall apart? How long will they hold up psychologically? How long will they hold up physically?

How many nights in succession, and how many times per night, can Aunt Elinda declare a state of emergency, and wait tensely with bags packed and escape route planned in order to ensure the safety of an eight-year-old little girl before the child starts to react defensively against the constant psychological strain?

And what if there were no crashing thunder and flashing lightning? What if the bombs never fell? What if the boy's warning cries about the wolf had everything to do with his desire to feel important and nothing to do with real wolves?

Then the declared state of emergency would be based on lies and trickery. That would hardly improve the public mood.

When a state of emergency is declared the adrenaline starts to pump, and with adrenaline levels high enough people are capable of committing murder for much less than having their night's sleep disturbed.

You have certainly heard your neighbors complain. *Some of us have to get up and work tomorrow. We need our sleep!*

And now your infant is complaining...

And she has every right to because not only have you declared a permanent state of emergency through your constant *rescue efforts* – affix the labels safety, intimacy or comfort if it amuses you, but rescue efforts are what they are – you have also been less than truthful.

The wolf is *not* at the door.

The bed is *not* dangerous.

The wolf is NOT going to take your child.

That is the truth. And it will remain so unless things change, but let's not go there.

The truth is: *You can rest easy. We are watching over you. We know the danger and we will keep it at bay. Your survival is guaranteed.*

If and when you decide to embark upon the *Good-Night's-Sleep Cure*, that is the *truthful*, satisfying message you will convey to your child – and you will do so in a way that your *child* finds convincing.

And I can promise you that your only regret in all this will be that you didn't apply the *Good-Night's-Sleep Cure* sooner!

The results will be as peerless as they are certain.

3. ENJOYMENT

Young children should be enjoyed – and enjoy themselves!

Little Leonard's mother writes:
Our Leonard is now 18 months old and the pride and joy of the whole family. His parents especially of course.

Just over a year ago, we were unfortunately less clued in to our little boy's way of expressing himself. I was lost. No one was sleeping! At least three times an hour, we would feed him and lug him around, and we thought that it all would sort itself out.

Finally, I'd had enough. I realized that our family – the whole family – needed to sleep. I surfed the net and found the Good-Night's-Sleep Cure. *I read until my eyes were square and 24 hours later, we started the cure. After one week, we had a home run.*

This has meant the world to us. We hadn't understood Leonard. I didn't know how to listen. Anna Wahlgren enabled me to crack the code.

My husband can now entertain the idea of having another child. A year ago, the prospect was less than tempting. We were dead on our feet.

Since my philosophy is 'Hope for the best, but prepare for the worst', I have been expecting some kind of relapse over the last year, but it hasn't happened. Leonard is beautiful, smart, fun and generally adorable, and we are A HAPPY FAMILY!

Thanks, Anna! You have helped us become the parents that Leonard deserves.

If and when you decide to embark upon the *Good-Night's-Sleep Cure*, and after you have patiently and diligently read the whole book – preferably until your eyes are bloodshot – you will have come to realize that this cure is more than a sleep strategy. It is a philosophy of living.

It's about enjoying life, enjoying a good sleep, enjoying good food, enjoying being a part of the common struggle for existence, enjoying the dawn of each new day and the dusk that signals each day's end, enjoying good cheer, music and laughter, enjoying peace and tranquillity, enjoying good will and friendship, enjoying the beauty that is so abundant on this earth in nature, people, plants and animals, enjoying being alive, enjoying loving and being loved. It's about enjoying the act of enjoying!

If you are wondering who those words are intended for, you or your child, the answer is both of you.

You are both human beings. Admittedly, one of you is big and one of you is little, but you are both made of flesh and blood in God's image.

Infants are made of exactly the same stuff as we adults.

You recognize yourself in your child. Doesn't he have your nose? Doesn't she have your eyes? Aren't his dimples exactly like yours? Doesn't she have your curls? And what about body type? Don't you look for some talent or other that your child must have inherited from you? Don't you spot some personality trait that can only be traced back to you?

The *Good-Night's-Sleep Cure* will enhance your recognition abilities to the extent that you will be able to discern what you and your child have in common just by virtue of belonging to the human species.

The basic human need for *food, sleep and security* is something you, your child and every other living being share.

Having searched so desperately for the help you need to sleep through the night, you can now see that your young child is actually doing the same thing.

You would give your right arm for a sound, undisturbed night's sleep, something you took for granted before you had children. You can now understand that your child, if she could choose, would happily return to the womb and the blissful peace that reigned before birth.

You know from your own experience what an effective torture technique sleep deprivation is, so you can see your child's sleep deprivation for the wolf that it is.

You have had to manage on short, fitful naps whenever you could grab them.

Your child has too.

But the price has been high. Too high. Your family life is threatened, as is your professional life and your love life... You have no energy. You can't function.

That is just how your child feels.

You have only functioned for as long as you have because you *had* to function. You have to take care of all the basic necessities. You have to *hold out*. But deep down you believe that there ought to be more to life than just *holding out*.

You don't just want to survive. You want to live!

So does your child.

In a nutshell, both you and your child want to *enjoy* what life has to offer.

With the *Good-Night's-Sleep Cure* at the back of your tired mind, you will never again think that the need for sleep places a strain on your child.

Sleep is a gift from God, and the most natural thing in the world for every human being, big or small, is sleeping at night. It's a blessing to quietly pray for: a sound, long, undisturbed, secure sleep!

It is a delight.

If and when you embark upon the *Good-Night's-Sleep Cure* and apply it properly with *peace* as the foundation and *security* as the supporting pillars, your child will crown the edifice with *enjoyment* all by herself and will take liberating flight into a starry firmament of boundless possibilities.

As you see, it is easy to wax lyrical about enjoyment. But I think you agree with me. Your nights will soon be your own again, and how you will enjoy them! How you will enjoy your meals when you are no longer sad and exhausted but can eat with a lusty appetite! How you will enjoy your beloved, your long neglected friends, your interests and hobbies. How you will enjoy music, joyous laughter, work and life!

And that is exactly what infants who are at long last able to sleep do. They *enjoy* their sleep and all the other good things in life.

How does this enjoyment manifest itself? What actually happens?

As early as the second and third nights, when you lay the foundation of the *Good-Night's-Sleep Cure* with *peace*, you will see the first signs of the approaching enjoyment.

- Your child will begin to listen to your jingle and believe you.
- Your child will begin to fall back to sleep by herself between ever fewer wakeful periods without your even having to jingle.
- Your child will be eating with a hearty appetite by the third day. (We will talk more about how the cure affects the child in the next chapter.)

And you? Will you dare think you see a light flickering forlornly on the horizon? Indeed you might, as you sit on the sofa with your partner after a bedding procedure that has taken all of two minutes. You might find yourselves asking each other, 'So what shall we do tonight?'

During the follow-up week, when you strengthen the supporting pillars of *security* and do it in a way that completely convinces your *child* that this is a structure built to last, your child will respond by sleeping through the night for the first time in her young life. Twelve hours, eleven, eleven and a half – whatever you have decided.

And what about you?

Now it will begin to dawn on you that the vicious cycle of sleep deprivation, lack of appetite, debilitating exhaustion and dull indifference to just about everything is about to be broken. Is it possible that you will be able to sleep through the night? And have your evenings free? If the answer is yes, then endless vistas open up! You can actually do things. How about starting with a gourmet dinner, just the two of you? When was the last time you and your partner indulged yourselves in such a delight?

And then, once you find yourselves able to count on actually being able to sleep at night because your child does, you will enter the so-called zombie stage. This can last anything from one to two weeks, during which time you will sleepwalk your way through life.

Your friends may say, 'You can sleep now. Why are you so tired?'

'Because we can sleep,' is the proper response.

Imagine an exhausted, stressed out workaholic who is on call 24-7. He hasn't seen hide nor hair of his family for a whole year. He finally has the chance to go on a two-week vacation with them. Everyone is just going to kick back, smell the flowers and enjoy the reunion. What would he do? Sleep like a log. He would sleep the entire vacation away! He wouldn't have the strength for anything else. He wouldn't even give his disappointed mother the time of day. He wouldn't have the strength to play with the kids. He wouldn't be able to summon the energy to engage his partner in some much needed amorous activities. He would do absolutely nothing. Except *sleep!*

The zombie period is a quasi-conscious time for recovery. It is the down period that precedes enjoyment. Our exhausted workaholic needs six weeks' vacation, not two.

And your child? Once she has been helped to find the *peace* to relax and the *security* to sleep at night, she will get sick!

Nine times out of ten, children develop some kind of fever as soon as they get the opportunity to release what they have been holding back for so long. Rather like the workaholic on vacation.

But later, after the parents' zombie period and the child's sick period, everyone's batteries are recharged. Then a positive cycle has been established. Then it's full speed ahead for *enjoyment* on all fronts and by everyone involved.

An important part of the *Good-Night's-Sleep Cure* is the *laugh-before-bed*.

You have probably been told that putting infants to bed should be preceded by so-called gradual de-escalation. The day must wind down. Silence must descend, the lights must be dimmed, bed-time stories must be read but in a low voice. The parent(s) must coo all the way to the edge of the child's bed and preferably lie down with the child themselves, stroking and patting her until she falls asleep.

There is a subliminal message that infants who have to sleep at night should somehow be pitied. (Their loving parents, who aren't *allowed* to sleep at night are to be pitied too.) The slow de-escalation, which often takes hours, supposedly paves the way for drowsiness. Children have to *want* to take the sleep they need, and they are supposedly capable of taking the sleep they need. And this they cannot do before they are really tired. Or ready to pass out. Thus, they have to be tired out properly.

The *Good-Night's-Sleep Cure* argues in favor of another approach.

Infants should be put to bed in good time, and they should be put to bed when they are really happy!

Young children should laugh before they sleep. Ideally, they should laugh all the way to bed. Before they go to bed or are put to bed, they should have the time of their young lives. They should laugh until they can barely breathe. If nothing else works, then tickle them, but laugh they must.

Why?

Put yourself in their place. You have had a hard, dreary, uninspiring, completely meaningless day. If you had to go to bed in the frame of mind that you are in, without so much as a glimmer of good cheer over the last twelve hours, you would hardly be looking forward to the day that awaited you when you woke up. You would probably draw out going to bed in the hope that something would happen to make the day at least marginally worthwhile. You would try to have fun during the evening and experience something positive, meaningful or simply beautiful so that there would have been some *point* to it all. Then you could go to bed with something to feel good about and with renewed confidence. You might even be able to look forward to the next morning!

That is exactly how young children function. They also have days when nothing goes right. That can be caused not least by overtiredness, something that builds up over months (perhaps years) in children who suffer from sleeping difficulties. You can relate to this from your own experience. If you are constantly tired, life loses its lustre.

That is why young children should have a rollicking good time before they sleep, whether they want to or not, I would argue. They should laugh loud and long. Reading stories, cuddling, coochie-coochie-cooing, should be scheduled for earlier in the day. It should not be a part of the evening procedure, when *having fun* should top the agenda.

After the bedtime laugh, the bedding procedure itself shouldn't take longer than two minutes.

The subliminal message isn't that sleeping is stressful for young children. The message here is exactly the opposite. Children who are allowed to sleep are no more to be pitied than their loving parents.

Sleeping at night is as obviously natural as it is obviously necessary for big people as well as little ones. Furthermore, it is delightful and desirable!

The bedtime laugh emphasizes that sleeping at night is *positive*. It's great fun to go to bed/be put to bed. It's party time!

The bedtime laugh throws the door to *enjoyment* wide open.

Towards the end of the follow-up week or the week after that at the latest, when you have followed all the provisions of the *Good-Night's-Sleep Cure* to the letter, you will see that this is true.

Then you will see how your young child, who, let's say, isn't walking yet, crawls off to her crib and stretches out her arms towards it. She will look at you, her loving parents, who have been putting on an Oscar winning performance to amuse her, with a look that says, 'You two are really funny and it's been great, but please, can one of you lift me up to bed now so that I can *sleep?*'

This is the experience that awaits you every evening, once you have properly administered the cure. Your child will sigh with delight at the prospect of sleeping in her bed in the (now) relaxing darkness with her teddy bear or whatever she has appointed her toy-friend, under her comfortable blanket, undisturbed, *secure* and at peace.

If you insist on hanging around in your child's designated sleeping space, you run the risk of being unceremoniously kicked out.

And that is not a particularly appealing thought: that you can be perceived and actually *be* a nuisance. It's not easy for a conscientious mother to accept that she is not always God's only gift to her child. *Mommy's here. Now everything will be fine!*

If mother disturbs her child's sacred sleep, something is amiss. Her child will reject her in one way or another. Older children will simply tell her like it is. '*Go away!*' Mother will then have to swallow her pride and bear in mind that she doesn't like anyone invading her sleeping space at night either.

And you will also experience what perhaps is the greatest delight of all: your child will greet each new day with a song and greet you with a smile so bright it will eclipse the sun.

Now we are not talking about well-being. We are talking about *enjoyment.*

And that is where you will eventually arrive, if and when you decide to embark upon the *Good-Night's-Sleep Cure.* That is the destination you will give your child the prerequisites to reach.

Don't be content with anything less.

Your child shouldn't have to be content with anything less!

I have used the word *liberating.* I described your child's delight over a sound, secure, peaceful sleep as a *liberating flight into a starry firmament* from the edifice – the philosophy of living – that is the *Good-Night's-Sleep Cure.*

Let me explain:

If you were starving to death, all your thoughts, your entire consciousness, would revolve around laying your hands on food. The instinct to survive is the most powerful instinct we have.

If you are hungry, your larder is empty, the grocery store's shelves are empty of everything except dust, you have no money, and you have no idea where your next meal is coming from, you would hardly be interested in love, comfort, clean clothes and tenderness.

Physical imperatives are what count under such circumstances and the most urgent of them all is survival. You would not be able to think about anything else.

And once you found food in sufficient quantities to get through *that* day, your thoughts would immediately turn to the problem of laying your hands on food to get you through the next. Before you *knew* you were going to survive, you wouldn't be able to relax. You would be incapable of focusing on anything else.

You would transform yourself into a less than free person.

Unless you knew that the physical, practical prerequisites for survival were guaranteed, you would not be able to take your place on the school bench of life, educate yourself, develop, grow and realize your potential in accordance with A. H. Maslow's axiom, *'What a man can be, he must be.'*

When people are starving, they hunt for food and nothing else.

Similarly, shackled by sleep deprivation as you are, you are unfree. You know it depletes you and breaks you down. Everything that was once important to you, everything that was fun, stimulating, educational and enriching has faded into pallid, futile illusions. You can barely remember what it feels like to actually *want* to do something. The only thing you want to do is sleep at night. That overshadows everything.

Sleep deprivation has taken over your life. And you know very well that your need for sleep, undisturbed sleep, sufficient sleep and predictable sleep – sleep you can *count on* – transcends the physical. If it didn't, you wouldn't be on the edge of a breakdown, and sleep deprivation would not be the effective method of torture that it is.

If human beings are unable to satisfy their most basic needs – the need for food, sleep and security – they become locked in a vicious cycle of survival anxiety that is impossible to break out of.

If their basic needs are partially met every now and then, they will manage. If they are strong, they will manage just fine. They can, at least occasionally, rise above the law of the jungle, whose prime directive is survival at any cost.

But they are still unfree. They are still shackled. They may not be bound hand and foot, but they have a sizeable ball and chain to drag behind them. They are never truly free of anxiety, insecurity and a devastating feeling of vulnerability, no matter how successful they are at suppressing their survival anxiety. Spreading their wings takes tremendous courage. Just *holding out* consumes all their time and energy.

Once their basic needs are generously satisfied, not just after the fact when they have become acute, but *preventively*, continuously and with a comfortable margin, then they can soar to the stars.

Then they are free to develop their full human potential.

Then they are free, the opposite of bound, shackled and unfree.

You child will become a living illustration of this, if and when you embark upon the *Good-Night's-Sleep Cure* and see it through to that goal that is called *enjoyment*.

Enjoying life is a liberating aria that breaks chains that bind her to the earth.

Your child's development will literally explode under these conditions. You will not need to 'coach' or 'stimulate' it. *What a man can be, he must be!*

'*Leonard is beautiful, smart, fun and generally adorable, and we are A HAPPY FAMILY!*'

You will be able to sign off on these words, and substitute your own child's beautiful name.

Young children should be enjoyed – and enjoy themselves!

THE CHILD AND THE CURE
4 MONTHS TO 12 YEARS

Young children do not have to be burdened with sleep problems. Or, more accurately, well-meaning parents do not have to burden their children with sleep problems.

But it's easy to do. You have no doubt noticed by now that you are not the only parents who are not permitted to sleep at night. Sleep problems are by far the greatest worry among the parents of infants and young children today (2009). The very term 'sleep problem' raises the question of definition, but the great majority of all children from six months to pre-school age do *not* sleep twelve hours a night. They sleep far less, and, to make matters worse, they wake up two to three times a night. There are statistics that confirm this.

You may have been given the impression that everyone else's children sleep better than yours. That's because parents are not keen on admitting how bad things actually are.

And this in turn is due to the fact that all parents, deep down, know that young children need to sleep at night. They blame themselves, just as you do I'm sure, because 1) they can't get their kids to sleep so they are bad parents and 2) they are cracking under the strain of their own unbearable sleep deprivation, which makes them even worse parents. If only they were saints. Saints don't need to sleep.

Everyone beautifies the truth a touch. 'He sleeps just fine. Wakes up every now and then, but it's not a problem.'

If and when you embark upon the *Good-Night's-Sleep Cure* and follow it meticulously, with *peace* as the foundation, *security* as the supporting pillars, and *enjoyment* as the edifice's glistening crown, visible for the world to see, even for those who don't see that well, the naked truth will out. People will stop beautifying the truth about their catastrophic nights. They will tell it like it is. 'We're going crazy! We can't take another night! How did you do this?!'

A US study claims that three out of four parents want to improve their children's sleeping habits. At the same time, 90% of parents say that they *think* their children sleep enough.

It has been demonstrated that infants, young children, school children, and teenagers do not sleep enough. Children of all ages sleep on average one hour less than they did 30 years ago. (It is 47 years since I had my first child, and if we go back that far, I think we can add another hour; back then children slept on average *two* hours more than they do today.)

That hour (or those hours) confirms that children and adolescents suffer from chronic sleep deprivation. This takes its toll on their brains, which are sensitive and continue to develop up until the early 20s. There are a number of researchers today who see a catastrophic connection between sleep deprivation, perceptual abilities, concentration, memory and emotional stability. Chronic sleep deprivation during the sensitive years of childhood and adolescence can result in permanent neurological damage. This damage is not a hangover that can simply be slept off and it may contribute to stress, depression, compulsive eating, child obesity, ADHD and suicide.

That is why I think parents in the Western World should wake up to the reality that the 'truths' they have been fed – that children don't need that much sleep, that children take all the sleep they need, that wakeful nights resulting in too little sleep for all concerned are the parents' problem not the child's – are in fact a pack of lies.

It's time to admit the folly of our ways!

Children need to sleep at night. They need twelve hours a night until they are well into their school years. Period.

It wasn't my own children that motivated me to develop the *Good-Night's-Sleep Cure.* It was other people's.

Everything I know about young (and not so young) children, I have learned first hand. Kids have been my university.

I have lived and worked with children my entire adult life. I have never worked outside the home. I knew nothing about babies when I had one of my own at nineteen. I had no idea what I was doing. I had not grown up in a family, so I didn't have much to draw on. I was forced to try to learn from my *child.*

My starting point was that the kid was probably made of the same stuff I was.

And she was. Like me, she was a human being of flesh and blood with the same basic needs.

What I learned from her was *human universals.* Her eight siblings, the youngest of whom is now 30, further educated me on the subject.

God has given me a the gift of being able to *understand* young children, just as He has given some people a knack for understanding horses (definitely not one of my talents) and equipped others with green fingers (ditto). Thus, my first child was not an experiment. I observed her with curiosity and a willingness to learn, and I had an uncanny ability to see things from her side of the fence, something I can only thank my Creator for.

I acted in accordance with *her* questions and reactions, rather than the dictates of the conventional wisdom of the time.

Forty-seven years ago, the four-hour principle was all the rage. A baby should be breastfed every four hours. After the meal – which was to last no more than 20 minutes – both breasts should be completely emptied. Breast pumps were not to be had in maternity wards, where mothers spent the first week after giving birth and were confined to their beds for the first three days. They had to pump out their milk by hand. By the third day the milk was flowing and only then was the baby delivered for feeding. There was none of this 'rooming-in' stuff.

Once home, the baby was to have a specific amount of milk at each feeding. There were tables indicating how many grams should be given at what age. The rations were stingy I soon learned, but weight gains were monitored by the local children's clinic. If the baby gained 200 grams a week, all was well.

In order to ensure that their babies were getting the requisite number of calories, new mothers were encouraged to rent a scale. Babies were to be weighed before and after every meal. I remember that 110 grams of milk per meal was the standard ration for a four-week-old infant.

At the one-month mark, babies were to be weaned off the night feeding (singular in those days). Cradles were mandatory. To quiet babies down, their carriages could be drawn back and forth over thresholds and carpet edges. Rides in cars with the baby in a carry cot were also recommended. Very progressive in a time when not everyone owned a car! Baby seats and seat belts had not yet appeared.

And as soon as the stump of the umbilical cord had fallen off together with its gruesome clip, babies could be put down on their stomachs. 'Frog sleeping' it was called. Until then, babies were put down on their sides in the fetal position with a rolled up blanket at their backs. Alternating sides was the only requirement.

Against this backdrop, I arrived home with my one-week-old baby, and did exactly as I had been told. But my baby just screamed. And screamed. And screamed.

Why was she screaming? According to the scales and the tables, she was getting everything she was supposed to, so why wasn't she happy? She screamed round the clock. You, dear reader, probably understand that, short though that sentence is, it conjures up enough blood, toil, tears and sweat to drown a continent.

I had the incredible good luck to discover after two weeks at home that there was something wrong with the scales we had rented. My baby hadn't been getting what she needed. She had *lost* weight since her birth.

So I threw tables and scales to the four winds and devoted myself exclusively to my baby's well-being. She was fed until milk was virtually coming out of her ears. The screaming stopped immediately and never resumed.

The following week, she did nothing but eat and sleep, eat and sleep. Then she celebrated her return to the living with her first magnificent smile.

I say incredible good luck because it resulted in a parting of the ways. It wasn't the children's clinic's fault that the scales were defective, but scales that worked subsequently showed that when my baby was allowed to eat until she was full to bursting, she was chowing down almost twice the ration that the children's clinic recommended.

And this continued throughout the first year. If she was allowed to eat until she was full, really full, at every meal, she didn't scream. She *enjoyed life*.

I didn't understand why the recommended rations were so cheap. Why was it necessary for infants to be placed on a starvation diet? *Make sure you don't give her too much to eat* was the constant refrain. I didn't tell the truth of course. I didn't just give her as much food as she could get down in 20 minutes, but stuffed her with appetizer and dessert for at least 20 minutes more – at every single meal.

Not long after that I heard colic discussed for the first time. Chilling tales of infants who screamed day and night for three months abounded.

Since I had learned to think for myself, thanks to the defective scales, I knew what had transformed my little fog horn of a baby into such a quiet, contented little soul: food, lots of food, more food and still more food. I ruminated on my own theory concerning colic. And it would be field-tested and validated hundreds of times in the coming years: *colic is unalleviated survival anxiety.*

Children are not born with colic. No child is predestined to develop colic, just as no woman is predestined to get headaches and no man is predestined to have ulcers.

But my prescription – food, lots of food, more food and still more food – has resulted in countless children being cured, once their parents tossed out the tables and stuffed their babies so full of food it was running out both ends.

For the first time – but not the last – I wondered over the bizarre contention that babies should feel only moderately well. They should feel more or less all right, but don't go overboard! They should eat as much as they need, but no more. They should sleep as much as they need to, but no more. (That was permitted in those days, unlike now – but letting them scream themselves to sleep was just fine. That much hasn't changed.)

Infants should not wallow in well-being was the rule, then as now. They should not *enjoy* life. They should cry and have problems.

And above all, they should cause problems, not least for their loving mothers.

Perhaps there is a connection between the women's movement and the market's insatiable need for labor. As early as the beginning of the 1960s, it was très a la mode to regard young children as a tiresome hindrance to just about everything.

Suspicious person that I am, I sensed a sociopolitical conspiracy. Children were *supposed* to be tiresome. It made it easier for mothers to disengage themselves.

Throughout the 1970s, the public debate was dominated by complaints, not just about children, but about the family as an institution. Divorce rates soared and these new divorcees angrily demanded that society care for and raised their young children.

Children subjected women to a frightful ordeal. It was difficult to be pregnant with them, difficult to give birth to them, difficult to look after them, and difficult to get rid of them. There weren't enough day-care spots for everybody.

My little girl was happy. She was as contented as a little person could be – or a big one for that matter. She ate like a horse, slept like a log, *worked* with gusto and met the world head-on like the fearless explorer that she was (and remained) with an intellect that sparkled like the Milky Way.

Was she happy because she had her mother at home?

I wouldn't go that far. I never overestimated my importance as a caregiver on a personal level. My little girl didn't even call me 'Mom' because I never referred to myself in such terms. I was Anna. My ambition was to be available as her best friend in all the world. I was an ally who looked out for her interests, which of course she was incapable of doing herself.

My input consisted of giving her the *prerequisites* for her own development, development that evolution had hard wired her for.

It didn't take me long to figure out that if her development was to be given the free rein it deserved – *what a man can be, he must be* – she had to eat more than what was required for mere survival, and she had to sleep more than the minimum necessary for her to 'manage' on.

As has already been said, when a little person – or a big one – has her basic human needs satisfied with a comfortable margin, not just after the fact when the shortfall has become acute, but *preventively*, continuously and generously, then she is free to soar to the stars. Then she is free to develop her full human potential. Then she is truly free – as opposed to being bound, shackled and unfree.

'You must never have a moment to yourself' people sighed sympathetically when my daughter turned one. I didn't really understand what they were talking about. Did they feel sorry for me? Why?

I had as many moments to myself as I needed. Actually, I had hours. My child slept twelve hours a night. She played by herself in her crib for two hours every morning, devoting herself to pedagogical problem solving (and occasionally took a little nap). She slept for one and a half hours in the afternoon and was put to bed by her dad at six in the evening. What did I have to complain about?

I understood that I *should be* complaining. If I had told the truth, which was that I could hardly wait to *enjoy* this happy, clever, endlessly interesting little person's company during the time that I *didn't* have to myself, it would have fallen on deaf ears.

I think you know where I am going with this. Young children should be enjoyed – and enjoy themselves!

Anything else is indefensible, whatever the conventional wisdom says.

But today, almost half a century later, this conventional wisdom still holds sway, and since I am as suspicious now as I was back then, I still regard it as a conspiracy. Young children are difficult and must *remain* so. It creates employment for so many people. It has given birth to a vast industry with countless subsidiaries, each hawking a wide variety of products and 'services'.

What would the world be like if it were inhabited by harmonious youngsters who felt great, enjoyed being alive, and uninhibitedly used their healthy, well-developed brains? Who would be able to oppress *them*?

Today, it is sleep deprivation that condemns the young – and the not so young – to physical, spiritual and intellectual *unfreedom*.

Young children's sleep problems did not just fall out of a clear blue sky. Our culture *cultivates* them. Children are not born with sleep deprivation, just as they are not born with colic.

According to my conspiracy theory, not only have well meaning parents in the developed world acted against their better judgment and not satisfied their young children's basic human needs in a way that satisfies their *children*, they have actually been set up to fail.

And that is why the *Good-Night's-Sleep Cure* is viewed as controversial by so many of the powers that be (although not by children).

The *Good-Night's-Sleep Cure* does not content itself with helping young children sleep just enough but no more so that their parents can sleep just enough but no more. The *Good-Night's-Sleep Cure* aims high. It aims for *freedom* – freedom for everyone, big and small!

If you don't know what I am talking about, you most certainly will once you have seen the *Good-Night's-Sleep Cure* through to its wonderful conclusion. Your child will show you exactly what I mean with all the luminous clarity you could desire.

Mental freedom first requires physical well-being!

At three weeks, once her stomach was full to bursting, my baby slept six to seven hours at a stretch with no help other than peace and quiet. From one month on, this is the rule rather than the exception for infants *who are given as much food as they can take on board and then some at regular intervals during the day.*

In connection with the true birth, which takes place at the end of the second week of life or the beginning of the third, '*and then some*' takes on crucial significance.

Still larger rations are required towards the end of the second month.

If that little tummy is more than full, a two-month-old will happily allow the nights to be extended to eight hours. A little calming may be required at the beginning, but not much. A two-month-old – under the right circumstances – will prove herself to be a grateful creature of habit.

At three months, a ten-hour night can be introduced and at four months, a twelve-hour night.

And since this makes the Cure unnecessary, you can give *A Good Night's Sleep* to someone who needs it more!

There are several reasons that I recommend the *Good-Night's-Sleep Cure* for fussy little sleepers from precisely four months. (There is no upper limit as we will soon see.)

- The jingle has more effect on a four-month-old than younger infants, since younger babies will try to connect to a face.
- Healthy four-month-olds of normal weight are perfectly capable of sleeping soundly for twelve hours without being fed.
- The need to suck has diminished substantially. A four-month-old has no need for a pacifier, whether of the artificial or natural variety.
- Four-month-olds can turn over, not only from stomach to back but also from back to stomach, which gives them the freedom to choose the position they prefer.
- Last but not least, it takes time to create a situation so chaotic, desperate and sleep-deprived that the parents can't stand it anymore. A four-month-old who has been shackled to the ball and chain of survival anxiety ever since the exodus from the womb can't stand it anymore either. *This far and no further* goes for all concerned. It is not only the parents who are seeking help. The child in her chaotic state is seeking help too. If anyone thinks that four-month-olds, by their own initiative, will sleep better

tonight, tomorrow night, or the night after that, that hopeful illusion is quickly shattered by the babies themselves. Since you have read the chapters on *Peace, Security* and *Enjoyment,* you know why.

Four months
Lottie, who describes herself as 'a very happy mother', writes:

I just had to tell you that the Good-Night's-Sleep Cure *has produced stunning results in my four-and-a-half-month-old baby. I administered the cure with the baby on her back and it worked out brilliantly. I am so happy! Thank you!*

PS. We have just gotten home from a four-day vacation, and I can report that the follow-up week went brilliantly too, in spite of an unfamiliar environment, an unfamiliar carriage and an unfamiliar bedroom.

Young children do as they are taught.

You might say that a newly arrived baby behaves just as we would at a new workplace.

First we get settled. Then we familiarize ourselves with our duties. We have our supervisors and co-workers to help us, and we have our education and experience. We learn a lot by watching what other people do.

Babies lack experience. They learn by watching others and by leadership.

A human child is born to explore, master and eventually change her reality, her living conditions, and her world.

For a child to be able to explore, master and change reality, that child must be presented with the reality that reigns whether the child is around or not.

A new employee can only learn to perform his duties successfully if a functioning enterprise exists.

Few people begin a new job without knowing something about what the job entails. But not even the most qualified new employees would try to remake the work place and toss out all the work routines on their first day on the job.

An infant who changes the 'work place' just by existing and finds the routines have been trashed or never introduced in the first place will react with anxiety, confusion and dissatisfaction.

Young children do as they are taught. Your child follows your lead and learns from you whether you like it or not.

If you follow your child's lead, however, your child will lose no time in protesting, just as you or I would if, on our first day on the job, the CEO laid responsibility for running the company on our shoulders.

That is precisely the predicament that little four-month-old Adam, our candidate for the cure, finds himself in.

Adam refuses to accept responsibility for the Company. This refusal was evident already at two months, when he sought but didn't find a well-structured routine in his daily existence.

Now his refusal is becoming more and more stubborn. He demands *leadership* from the people in charge.

Adam wasn't born filled with longing for his mother, whom he finally had the opportunity to meet in real life, nor was he born with an innate curiosity about his father, who was standing there in the delivery room proud and expectant. His happy parents perhaps desperately wanted to believe that Adam had been longing for them as much as they had been longing for him. I dare say most parents in these emotionally individualistic times want to believe that.

But Adam, like all babies, was born a pragmatist. There were only two vital questions that concerned him:

- Who is going to look out for my interests in this world so that my survival will be guaranteed?
- What do I have to learn in this world so that one day I will be in position to take care of myself?

If we rephrase these vital questions in terms that new employees might use, these questions would sound something like this:

- Who is going to look out for my interests in this company so that I can hang on to my job?
- What do I have to learn in this company so that one day I will be able to strike out on my own and set up my own business?

At four months of age, fussy sleeper Adam has still not received a satisfactory answer to his first vital question. As far as he is concerned, it is high time to dump survival anxiety in favor of an enthusiastic plunge into vital question number two with all that it entails.

Adam wants a future!

He isn't here to survive hand to mouth, rescued and comforted temporarily. He's here to *live*. That requires more than a rescue in the here and now. A safe and secure tomorrow has to be guaranteed as well – and all the tomorrows after that with the accompanying secure wolf-free nights!

The *Good-Night's-Sleep Cure* gives him a convincing, *secure* answer to vital question number one. And little Adam is anything but reluctant. He wants nothing more than not to have to fear for his skin.

Adam gratefully accepts the schedules and the routines that are put in place under *confident leadership*.

Adam has absolutely no problem with the fact that suddenly everything right down to the smallest detail has changed because he isn't stupid. He immediately understands that this is something that is in *his* interests. He is finally receiving answers to the question he has been asking more and more aggressively of late. He is receiving answers that *he* thinks are satisfactory.

Adam's cries haven't been expressions of discontent. They have been questions. *Is the wolf coming for me?*

It is not difficult for him to accept these repeated convincing, and convinced, assurances that he can feel completely *secure*. The wolf isn't coming. Not now, not later, not ever!

Little Adam is tailor made for the cure because he is exactly four months old. He is so wonderfully open to *acquiring* habits. Note that I didn't say new habits because he has never had any before. He has no old habits to break or give up. That he would have been capable of doing too, but what is so marvelous is that a four-month-old baby really is a creature of habit. It's written into his DNA. These tendencies are clear in all children as young as two months, but at four months, the creature of habit really hits its stride. It is merely a question of gratefully accepting – which is exactly what Adam does. He reacts to the *Good-Night's-Sleep Cure* with unshakable relief.

But won't he miss the pacifier? That's a habit, isn't it?

No. It is not in Adam's interests to be silenced with a plug in his mouth when it is *security* he is asking about (and asking questions is something he needs to do). He will forget the pacifier faster than his parents will.

Adam has been eating several times a night all his short life. When his sleep problems reached their apogee, he was waking up and being placed at his mother's breast once an hour.

After the first night of the *Good-Night's-Sleep Cure*, during which he wasn't fed for eleven hours, he wasn't even hungry, much to his mother's surprise. He was tired!

Adam's Mom and Dad worked out the following schedule for him. They chose an eleven-hour night in order to make room for evening socializing between father and son. Three naps during the day total four and a half hours, which fulfill Adam's total sleep quota of 15.5 hours out of 24.

Meals during the day begin every third hour.

Good morning 7.00. Feeding from both breasts for one hour at the most
Morning nap: 1.5 hours 8.30 to 10.00
Second meal 10.00 to 11.00 at the latest. Pureed fruit and breast milk
Midday nap: 1.5 hours. 11.30 to 1.00
Third meal 1.00 to 2.00 at the latest. Vegetable puree and breast milk
Afternoon nap: 45 minutes: 3.00 to 3.45
Fourth meal 4.00 to 5.00 at the latest. Fruit puree and breast milk
Early evening nap: 45 minutes 6.00 to 6.45
Fifth meal breast milk, bath and goodnight laugh 7.00 to 8.00
Good night 8.00

Five and six months

Little Sebastian's mother describes her life before and after the cure:

Six months ago, I had an oh-so-sweet son during the day. He slept well, ate well and all was sweetness and light. But then night fell. I tried to get him to sleep in his own bed, but it only worked if I sat with him, rocked him, patted him and sang to him until he fell asleep, which could take 40 minutes. Then he would wake up 45 minutes later, and I'd have to start all over again.

Naturally, I didn't have the strength for this, so he was allowed to sleep with us, something we had been doing from the beginning during the second part of the night (which kept getting longer). Back then, it was cozy. That didn't last. It got to the point that Sebastian could only sleep if he used me as a giant pacifier. For all that he kneaded and scratched my breasts for milk, he would get angry if the milk actually started to flow. He wasn't hungry.

He bit and kicked me. I was a complete wreck. In my heart of hearts, I was, to say the least, jealous of everyone who had children who slept at night. I didn't begrudge them their good fortune, but I wanted to find the strength to work my way out of those horrible nights.

Finally, I had had enough. I immersed myself in the Good-Night's-Sleep Cure. *I began to understand what the cure was really about and how little was actually required of me.*

Once I had made up my mind, I didn't want to wait another day. We administered the cure over Christmas and New Year's!

We have had our setbacks and our ups and downs, but obviously it's been mostly up. After three weeks, everything had fallen into place. Now I have a son who sleeps from 7.45 at night until 7.45 in the morning no problem, just as he takes his naps as he should. The cure didn't meet my expectations, it SURPASSED them.

Finally, I have a life again. I no longer have to wonder when I will have the time and the energy to do whatever needs to be done (because I never knew when Sebastian would sleep). I can cheerfully promise to do whatever whenever because I know I will have the time when he is asleep and I know I will have the energy. I am slept out!

At the beginning, I was uncertain about the daytime sleep periods too. I didn't want to be forced to live my life around the little guy's naps. And I wasn't! He comes with me everywhere and sleeps in the carriage at the appointed time wherever we happen to be. What freedom!

Exhausted parents that manage to survive fractured nights for more than four months seldom make it past five. Sleep deprivation becomes too much to bear. They realize that if sanity is to be preserved, the status quo is no longer an option.

And they have given up hope. They no longer believe that by some miracle, their children will suddenly start sleeping through the night all by themselves. It is now that they ask for help if they haven't done so already.

Five and six-month-old little babies are the second largest group that I have cured personally over the years.

The largest group of fussy sleepers is the eight to nine-month-old crowd. Their parents, who have been staggering through life with the help of every imaginable emergency measure, can now see what extremis their children are in. They suffer along with their children, who are close to complete collapse due to a lack of that vital deep sleep. They now desperately seek help for their *children's* sake, whereas the parents of younger children are still desperate over their own situation.

Around the five-month mark, a young child's personality emerges like a butterfly emerging from its cocoon. Now she is not 'just' a baby – and certainly not a newborn – that you have in your care to look after in the best way possible. From now on, you are dealing with an individual, a full-fledged little human being with distinctive personality traits.

It is a true metamorphosis!

We can now take the analogy we drew between a four-month-old and a new employee a little further.

Let's say a little five-month-old, Miss X, is beginning a highly skilled job at a company.

At first, her time is taken up with familiarizing herself with the new environment. Miss X doesn't know where her workstation is, nor does she know the names of her co-workers. She isn't even completely clear on what it is she will be doing. Her first few days on the job are stressful and she has a great deal to learn.

Finally, Miss X learns to find her way around the maze of corridors and gets a handle on her duties. She learns the names of her co-workers and figures out where they work and what they do. Life settles into a routine. Miss X earns herself a reputation as a resourceful employee and lives up to all her employer's expectations.

This is the stage that our four-month-old, creature of habit that she is, has reached.

But now things start to happen!

Miss X, who thinks that she knows what she needs to know about workplace routines, wants to improve herself. She decides she wants to know more about how the company actually works. She begins to see things in a larger context. She inspires the people around her and becomes bolder.

Miss X *is starting to think outside the box.*

This is the stage the five-month-old is at.

Miss X sallies forth as a personality in her own right, someone with ideas and a vision of the world, someone who knows what she wants to do and where she wants to go. She is no longer just a face in a crowd. Miss X stands out.

In just the same way, the five-month-old emerges from the crowd as a unique individual with a personality all her own and a soul that reaches for the heavens.

However, like us in our new workplace, if Miss X is to develop her personality, achieve her ambitions and follow her dreams – all in keeping with Maslow's axiom, 'What a man can be, he must be' – *physical and psychological freedom of manoeuvre* is required.

The two are inextricably linked, as we saw in the previous chapter. The generic term is simply *freedom:*

- When a human being – big or small – has her basic needs satisfied by a comfortable margin, not just after the fact when the need becomes acute, but *preventively*, continuously and generously, then she is free to soar to the stars.
- Then she is free to develop her full human potential.
- Then she is *free* as opposed to being shackled, bound and unfree.

Simply put, it's not just the loving parents who need to sleep at night!

Speaking of which, here is a little piece of gossip. When the parents of a five- or six-month-old child claim that their child's most prominent personality trait is a *strong-will*, I know that this is a family with sleep problems...

Without that innate and universal will power, the human species would have vanished from the earth a long time ago, so we should be grateful we have all been blessed with it.

It wasn't will power that caused a tiny fellow like Sebastian to scratch, bite, kick and knead his out-sized pacifier of a mother and turn her into a complete wreck. What he was expressing was pent-up *frustration*.

Mom had finally had enough, but little Sebastian, I would argue, had had enough long before that. He needed physical and psychological freedom to develop in accordance with the three points mentioned above.

He *demanded* it, and his mother was sensible enough to hear what he was trying to say.

With the help of the *Good-Night's-Sleep Cure*, she gave him his freedom. I have a feeling he has been showing his gratitude through his actions ever since!

A little Miss X by the name of Emma, just under six months old, came to me together with her dad to be cured.

Emma was tired when she arrived but apparently happy. However, her good cheer didn't last more than 20 minutes. Her parents then provided her with stimulation and entertainment, which ultimately only made her more tired.

Things have changed!

The sleep schedule that we put together, based on Emma's sleep requirements (15 hour and fifteen minutes/24) looked like this:

Night 8.00 to 7.00, 11 hours
Morning nap 8.00 to 8.45, 45 minutes
Mid-morning nap 9.45 to 10.30, 45 minutes
Mid-day nap 13.00 to 15.00, 2 hours
Late afternoon nap 17.00 to 17.45, 45 minutes

My notes from the first three nights (Dad took care of the fourth night and the follow-up week at home) provide a picture that is fairly typical of little Miss (and Mr) Xs.

Night 1

20.00   Dad puts Emma to bed and leaves. I buff and jingle. Emma falls asleep in 12 minutes.

22.15   Emma wakes up and asks. I buff and then jingle as I leave. She is tired. Buff and jingle, in and buff again, jingle as I leave, in and fan, jingle. She enjoys the buffing now!

22.32   Confirmation jingle + silence.

23.55   She wakes up again and asks. Buffing x 4 (ticked off when I stop). Jingle. Silence.

1.10   Asks again. A little buffing + jingle.

3.15   Wakes up, buffing + jingle, falls back to sleep at 3.17.

3.45   Jingle x 8. Buffing x 6 and jingle. Silence at 3.48.

5.15   New questions. Buffing x 4, jingle x 4. Silence at 5.18.

6.00   Wakes up very briefly, questions, buffing x 6 + jingle x 4.

6.20   Irritated. A little 'swearing'? A little buffing, jingle x 8.

6.25   Buffing. Jingle and confirmation. Silence at 6.30.

6.55   Surly, angry, tired. Buffing, jingle x 6. Silence.

7.05   Dad wakes her up happy-happy joy-joy.

Night 2

20.00 Dad puts Emma to bed. Buffs until Emma's little body relaxes. Quickly jingles his way out. I jingle x 4, combine reminder and confirmation. Emma falls asleep in 7 minutes.

21.17 Jingle x 4 (outside the door and away), silence at 21.18

3.55 Whine. Jingle outside the door x 4. Silence at 3.56.

4.03 Whine. Jingle x 4, pause, jingle x 4, pause, jingle x 8 (including confirmation), pause, jingle x 8 (4 somewhat irritated + 4 confirmation). Silence at 4.18.

4.57 Whine. Jingle x 6 (including confirmation), surly and confused reaction, whine, jingle x 6. Silence at 5.06.

5.07 Whine again. Quiets down by herself. Whine again. Quiets down by herself. I wait. Whine – jingle x 4. Has a small crisis and feels sorry for herself. She will have to take care of it. Confirmation when she is quiet at 5.12. New crisis, but she gets tired of it herself. Confirmation accepted. Silence.

5.15 Has second thoughts and starts up again. Quick buffing, quick fanning, exit jingle x 6 (including confirmation). Whine as soon as I stop! So I stop! Pause. Jingle x 8. Pause. Jingle x 8. (My voice is going!)

5.20 Buffing, fanning, OUT I think, jingle, wait outside, jingle again x 4. Wait.

5.28 Quick buffing, quick fanning, jingle my way out. Loud, angry crying. And presto! Silence at 5.31. Refrain from confirmation.

6.30 Jingle x 8 very loud. Silence. Whine. Jingle one last time x 6 including confirmation. Silence at 6.34.

7.00 Dad wakes Emma with great fanfare.

Night 3

20.00 Dad puts Emma to bed. No buffing because it's not necessary. Emma goes to bed cheerfully. Dad jingles and leaves.

20.45 She asks, but more whiney than anxious. I jingle. Loud, businesslike, firm. I wait. Very loud again x 4. Silence.

1.20 She hollers at the top of her lungs – and quiets down in 30 seconds. Gets sent on her way with confirmation jingle x 4.

5.40 Repeat of 1.20.

5.43 Repeat of 1.20.

5.47 Repeat of 1.20.

5.50 Go in and finish off with very short, very firm round of buffing (3 only), firm fanning pressure and out with jingle x 4. She quiets down during the jingle.

7.00 Dad wakes a sleepy girl with joyous acclamations and lifts her up in the air.

One month later, I received a report from Dad:

It is with great pride that I can tell you that Emma, now seven months old, sleeps like a princess every night without exception! How about that!

We have altered her schedule a little. It's the same as before, but we have taken away the afternoon nap. She gets a five-minute lie down if she wants. Then we put her to bed at 7.00 instead of 8.00. Now she gets 12-hour night, which she really likes.

During the day, she sleeps outside at least once. Works fine! We have also gotten her to take her two-hour nap indoors, which is good in the winter (brr).

Our other news is that she has gotten six new teeth in rapid succession, she has said 'mama' several times, and she is wriggling around earnestly trying to officially crawl!

Since I am an old lady now, I no longer cure children personally.

The problem with old ladies is that if they lose sleep at night, they can't make up the shortfall during the day. They can't even take three or four naps like normal five-month-olds. Life just isn't fair! Old ladies *have* to sleep at night or not sleep at all. Rather like most parents of infants I dare say.

So it is with relief – and tremendous joy of course – that I can state that the *Good-Night's-Sleep Cure* has stood the test of time and taken on a life of its own.

Others are taking over after me. Pioneering souls pass the wisdom on and it spreads like rings on the water. There is a grapevine linking parents and curers. I don't have to do anything except write this book!

But is it really possible to cure a child suffering from acute sleep problems with a *book?*

Yes, it is.

But is it possible to cure *twins* with a book?

That is possible too.

A letter from a Norwegian mother of twins:

Hi Anna,

First of all, I want to say that we are on night four of the cure of our six-month-old twin girls, the princesses Ingrid and Astrid.

They were one month premature and underweight (1.9 and 2 kilograms) and I breastfed day and night all summer. They soon got healthily chubby, but unfortunately they were used to being rocked, carried or nursed to sleep.

When they were five months old, I was being woken up about every two hours. I was lucky if I managed to square three hours of continuous sleep a night. Obviously, this was simply unsustainable.

I didn't know where I was going to get the energy to reverse the trend, and I didn't know how to go about it either. I refused to let them cry themselves into an exhausted sleep. NO WAY! (This method is recommended and widespread in Norway.)

It was my own mother who finally 'saved' me. She happened to be watching TV one morning (something she does very rarely) and caught an interview with you. She immediately told me about it. I liked what I heard and ordered your book via the net. I read it and was converted!

I decided to start in three weeks. I made up a schedule and forced my husband to read the book. He took a Friday off and on the Thursday evening, we started. We took one twin each, and each twin got her own room. We slept on camping beds in the hall.

The first night was somewhat chaotic for Astrid. (She was a hard nut to crack.

I think I must have jingled a hundred times, while I searched your book for more advice!)

We stuck to the schedule faithfully, even though it seemed a little cruel to wake babies who were so soundly asleep at the end of a 45 minute nap. But we would sing and clap our hands, and presto, they would smile at us with droopy eyelids.

To cut a long story short, we have succeeded beyond our wildest dreams. I can hardly believe it. I am expecting to be up occasionally during the wee small hours, but I have made your book my bible and I will stick to it.

Thanks so much for discovering this method!

Rest assured I will tell everyone I meet just how effective the Good-Night's-Sleep Cure *is for young children. As one of my girlfriends said today after I had told her that Ingrid had slept right through from 7 in the evening until 7 the next morning, 'You can take over from Anna Wahlgren now. You're young and you have a TON of excess energy'.*

'Yes,' I said. 'I can open up an AW subsidiary in Norway!'

I am so brimming with energy during the day (and evenings too, which start early now and not at 9.30) that I was able to write such a long letter to you about how down-to-earth and logical your method is. So once again, many thanks!

Marit, Jan Erik and our rosy-cheeked sleeping beauties, Ingrid and Astrid.

PS (one week later). The princesses are sleeping through the night and it takes two minutes to put them to bed, whether it's for the night or a daytime nap.

I never cease to be amazed at how simple it all is!

Eight and nine months

At between eight and nine months, a child's whole world is turned upside down. *The eight-month crisis* strikes.

What kind of an animal is sniffing around? A 'wolf' of course!

A young child this age can burst into tears at the mere sight of someone that she was happily babbling to the day before. Ensconced in Mom's arms this same child can desperately stretch her arms out towards Dad, which Mom finds both hurtful and ominous. Suddenly nothing makes sense!

Physical symptoms are many and varied: trembling, bizarre skin problems, fever and vomiting. The things children this age do to release tension are especially frightening. They have been known to bang their heads hard against the crib or the wall time after time.

Even kids who have always slept well and never needed the cure now often begin to wake up night after night. They cry piteously and show obvious signs of anxiety. The nights become fitful and ever more difficult to get through, and the parents are stunned by the lightning that has struck from a seemingly blue sky.

What is going on?

At between eight and nine months the 'I' is born. After nine months in mother's womb, the child comes into the world. After a similar period of time outside the mother's womb this child becomes 'I'.

This means that she becomes conscious of her own separateness. *I am my own person.*

I am someone. Mom is someone else. Dad is another someone else. I am not a part of them. I am me, distinct from them. The hands I use, my arms, my legs, my mouth, my knees, my body and my perceptions, all the tools I have at my disposal to live, all this taken together forms me. This 'I' is everything I think, feel and am.

When the 'I' is born, the child redraws all the boundaries. *I am no longer a part of the world that surrounds me.* I am in it and I belong to it, but I exist in it as a distinct entity, separate from it.

The child becomes conscious of this irrevocable disconnect.

Just as the physical birth approximately nine months ago was an almost traumatic event that changed everything for the child, the birth of the 'I' is an equally disorienting, transformative event.

Something irrevocable has happened, and the world will never be the same.

Thus, a child this age, who is no longer part of the surrounding 'space' but a separate entity located in this space, reacts like we all do when we journey into the unknown – with fear and uncertainty.

To understand how this transformative change is perceived by the child, we can draw a parallel with how a woman who has just given birth perceives her altered circumstances.

The child that has for so long occupied her womb is now outside her body, visible, palpable, very much in this world. This child is no longer part of her 'space'. Even though the mother-to-be knows that the child inside her has a life of its own, until it is born, it is a part of her.

Once born, the child is no longer a part of her in the same way. Forever removed from her body, the newborn lies at her breast, the umbilical cord cut. The child is still a part of her in that it is *her* child, but it is no longer a part of her body, even if this child, while it was inside her, was hers.

A loving, harmonious, companionable six to seven-month-old child who now, as an eight to nine-month-old, begins to fuss over anything and everything is reacting to a change just as dramatic as the change a woman experiences once she has given birth to her child.

Instability can appear in a child this age just as suddenly as it does in a new mother.

New mothers unanimously bear witness to how long it takes for them to wrap their minds around this profound change and adjust to it. A child going through the eight-month crisis also needs to reconcile herself and adjust to the change that takes place when the 'I' is born.

Unlike a grown woman, a child lacks the rationality that intellect confers. A child cannot say to herself, 'My I has been born. That's why everything feels so strange. Things will settle down soon. All the other babies who are going through the same thing say so.'

The woman, on the other hand knows. 'I have had a baby. That's why things feel so strange. I will get used to it.'

In the absence of rationality and experience, the child very easily falls prey to fear. The change that the child cannot relate to anything in her surroundings becomes terrifying.

And fear can manifest itself in countless ways. Outbursts directed at the immediate environment are not unusual. The 'I' has been born and the environment has therefore changed as well.

The birth of the 'I' requires a response, even if this response isn't *always* obvious.

Children this age, just like women who have recently given birth, react differently. In many children, the eight-month crisis manifests itself relatively gently. Nevertheless, the eight-month crisis is a time of instability. A new mother after all *is* unstable, regardless of whether or not it is noticeable and whether or not she suffers as a result.

And just like the new mother, a child whose 'I' has made its appearance adjusts to the changed circumstances more easily if daily life is simple and predictable and the surrounding environment offers warmth, peace and security.

Against this background, it is not hard to understand that a child who has given birth to her 'I' cannot be cured out of her eight-month crisis by her mother's attempts to lure her back to some kind of prolonged or renewed womb symbiosis. That would be as pointless as trying to cure a new mother of her undeniable physical and psychological instability by trying to put her baby back in her womb.

Separation anxiety, which psychologists never tire of discussing, has nothing to do with the mother. It has to do with what was old and familiar. It has to do with that which no longer is.

There's no going back, nor should there be – not for the mother who after the birth is no longer pregnant and not for the child who, eight to nine months later, will give birth to its 'I'.

Against this background, it is also not hard to understand that it is both rewarding and necessary to give fussy little sleepers going through the eight-month crisis the sound, secure sleep they so desperately need.

At eight to nine months of age, those children, who have never gotten the sleep they need either during the day or during the night throughout their short lives, are so exhausted that they show physical symptoms.

Now, if not sooner, the parents can usually see that their child is at the end of her rope. If the main problem thus far has been their own sleep deprivation, it is now that their *child's* sleep deprivation becomes glaringly obvious.

The child's skin is sickly pale, rather than rosy. Dark circles have settled under the eyes. The baby's eyes are blank and tired, rather than clear and expressive. She can barely keep herself upright and her little body often collapses like an accordion if she tries. Exhaustion hovers over her like a malign spirit. And people react. Things are not as they should be! That much is obvious for everyone with eyes to see.

And the fact that the situation is so unsustainable is what makes taking counter measures so rewarding.

Perhaps the results of the *Good-Night's-Sleep Cure* are at their benign best when the cure is administered to one of these sleep-deprived eight to nine-month-olds. There are several reasons for this.

- The children are so exhausted that they gratefully accept the help they finally get to find peace.
- The adult or adults who administer the cure do so in the firm belief that the *child* is the one who needs the help. They don't regard sleep as a strain on the child but recognize it for the vitally important and pleasurable asset that it is.
- Now there is no time to lose. The child has to be able to sleep. Giving up is not an option.
- Now as never before, it is clear that neither Mom nor anyone else can sleep for the child. This child has given birth to her 'I', and her sleep is her own.
- Peace and quiet, simplicity and predictability, and true security – this is the wish list for a child in the midst of the eight-month crisis. That internal agonizing changeability cries out for external steadfastness of purpose. And peace and quiet, simplicity, predictability and true security are exactly what the *Good-Night's-Sleep Cure* gives. Supply and demand meet in perfect equilibrium.

Little Hans, eight months old

For all practical purposes, little Hans didn't sleep at all. He managed the odd fitful couple of hours every now and then.

At the children's clinic, it was noticed that he didn't reach objects and grip them. It was suggested that he be given a neurological examination.

To enable him to sleep, the clinic wanted to give him 'tranquilizing drops' – a neuroleptic – which is about as tranquilizing as anesthesia.

His parents did not want him medicated. Nor did they want to believe that Hans had neurological problems.

When his mother came to me with a very tired little boy, Hans had just been given a walker. When he was placed in it, he had jumped up and down and looked happy.

He had also begun to pull himself up against various pieces of furniture – and tumbled over backwards to the floor. The children's clinic had recommended an indoor crash helmet (!).

Once the cure was completed, Hans' dad told his story in the guest book on my web page (www. annawahlgren.com, March 8 2003):

Hans was eight months old and he had always slept badly – if he slept at all. He didn't make up for the sleep he didn't get at night during the day. Sometimes we got the impression that he didn't sleep at all.

When we visited the local children's clinic, we always got the same answer when we asked why he wasn't sleeping. 'He is a social little guy who doesn't need to sleep. It's completely normal.'

Not being able to sleep is normal?

Since Hans was 'always' awake, our whole family was sleep deprived. Those short periods when Hans slept at night, we lay awake nervously and waited for him to wake up. We could never relax.

During one of my visits to the children's clinic, when Hans was eight months old, I was at wits end and I begged for help. Even if the people at the children's clinic hadn't been of much help up to now, I felt they were our last hope. If they couldn't help us, where were we supposed to go? I couldn't accept the standard answer, all that 'social little guy' stuff.

All I got out of them was a child psychiatrist's phone number. I could make an appointment with him and he could write out a prescription for Hans.

Before I left the clinic, the nurse mentioned in passing that she had heard that the writer, Anna Wahlgren, helps parents with kids who can't sleep, although she didn't sound too sure about it. In retrospect, it's kind of funny that it was the clinic that gave us information about Anna!

When I got home from the clinic and told my wife that we could choose between the psychiatrist and Anna Wahlgren, we weren't sure what we should do. Who could actually help us? How would we go about getting in touch with Anna? And would she want to help us? How could she get Hans to sleep when we have failed so abysmally for the last 8 months?

A few days later, I tried to phone Anna, but all I got was an answering machine. Frankly, I didn't expect her to return my call.

When I was in the car on my way home from work, Anna called and asked me a ton of questions. Her voice sounded so warm and cheerful. I told her about Hans and how worried we were about him. She then told me that of course she would help Hans, but there was no time to lose. She suspected that Hans was so tired that he must be feeling pretty lousy.

Just four days later, Hans and his mother went up to Anna's place in Gastsjon in the county of Jamtland, where they stayed three nights. We felt we had connected with someone who really knew what she was doing. And who wanted to help us.

When Hans came home after his sojourn in Jamtland, the little guy slept from approximately 6.30 in the evening to six the next morning. I couldn't believe it! Eleven and a half hours at one shot!

I was so overjoyed I didn't know whether to laugh or cry. I could hardly believe it was the same kid.

Next week Hans turns two, and he is still sleeping the sleep of the just. He is as happy as a lark during the day and hardly ever gets the blues. He loves his food and it's obvious how much he enjoys life. It's all thanks to Anna that Hans feels as good as he does. How would he be feeling if he hadn't gotten the help he needed?

It never ceases to amaze me there are still people in this stressed out world who *are willing to help others so tirelessly. As far as we're concerned, Anna is the patron saint of children!*

A little postscript from Dad in January 2005:
He is still sleeping wonderfully. Goes to bed around 7.00 and on weekends sleeps until 8.00 in the morning. We get up earlier during the week of course, since we both have to work. He doesn't always nap during the day, but more often than not he does. Eats like a horse.

Sleep and food spares us from illness and visits to the doctor. Incredible.

Hans has lots of little pals at day-care and among the kids in our neighborhood. He has a packed social calendar!

At the time of the cure, Hans was eight months old and after his fourth night at home, when he slept 11.5 hours at a stretch, he was placed in his walker again. He immediately got moving, his mother told me over the phone. He managed to propel himself the length of the large room all the way over to the stereo and energetically manipulated the buttons.

With the help of the walker, he could get around. Thanks to the height, he could reach the stereo. He had a clear goal. He would push the interesting buttons, turn the interesting dials and call forth – music! Four stages in a thought process in a little boy who until recently had been only been able to jump up and down on the spot a little in his walker – but who had looked happy.

He never again fell over backwards once he had raised himself up against something. He never needed that indoor crash helmet! And he could reach for things brilliantly and hold them in his hands for as long as he felt like it. He never needed that neurological examination!

There was nothing wrong with little Hans. He was just unbearably *tired.*

When Mom and Hans went home after their visit with me, I sent a letter to Dad with them. Here is an extract:

Thanks for lending me little Hans! He is a delightful little boy with a good head on his shoulders and a great interest in what goes on in the world!

He quickly understood what the drill was and he reacted – after an initial (and completely understandable) period of inflexibility – with obvious relief. On the second night, he slept nine and a half hours at a stretch – only to fall back to sleep.

I am glad he came. I don't think I'm exaggerating when I say that it was high time. During his short life, he had accumulated a sleep deficit that is not just unhealthy but flat out dangerous. It is not just burnt out adults that proliferate in Sweden today but, shockingly enough, burnt out infants.

Young children cannot 'work on autopilot' while their thoughts are a thousand miles away. They don't have the capacity to take mental holidays. They don't even have a frame of reference. Everything is strange, unfamiliar and difficult. Their concentration is total and it has to be. Their efforts to learn and understand are tireless and unceasing. Only sleep can – has to! – provide rest, recovery and renewed strength.

When you and his mother were trying to help him, comfort him and cheer him up, you were actually adding to his stress. You were disturbing him and making him terribly anxious. That is the bitter and paradoxical truth.

Every time you picked him up at night, you were doing him a disservice, pure though your motives were. Through your actions, you were confirming that the world was just as insecure and dangerous as he, in his worst bouts of survival anxiety, thought it was. You were saving him by protecting him with your bodies, which taught him that it is mortally dangerous to sleep without such protection.

The logic is simple: if all the measures you took to make him feel secure had been the right ones, he would have slept soundly.

The fact that I was able to break this vicious cycle in a single night makes it heartrendingly clear that the message he wanted and expected was that he could rest easy. The wolf wasn't coming for him. And he took that message to heart with great relief.

Once the routines settle and he knows in his bones that there are people – you, his loving parents – who are looking out for his interests, something which he by definition cannot do, you can see the difference in him; he is calmer, stronger, healthier, much happier and more evenly happy, and he no longer whines or cries.

By and large, Mom can explain the rest, but here are my instructions for the follow-up week:

1. *Perfect an appropriate, rhythmic goodnight jingle.*
2. *Let Mom 'buff' you and practice on her.*
3. *Stick to the schedule come hell or high water!*

A general rule is: Assume a leadership role.
In a nutshell, this is my rule of thumb:
A cry is a question, *not a complaint. This question requires* an answer, *not another question (which takes the form of insecurity).*

All newborn children know instinctively that they don't stand a chance of surviving on their own. They cannot obtain food, keep warm or protect themselves from the wolf. The instinct to survive is the counter weight to all this. The only possible result is survival anxiety. These children want to live, they have to live, but they believe and fear that they will die.

As a good caregiver and protector, you must do everything in your power to allay this anxiety as quickly and effectively as possible. This is done by constantly, through your actions, telling the child, 'You are going to survive. We will see to that. We are looking out for your interests. You can rest easy and devote yourself to living, growing, developing and having fun while you're at it! No wolf will get near you!'

This is the attitude that you should always have at the back of your head, an attitude that everything is completely, unequivocally self-evident.

'Should I really be lying here?' the child screams. 'Isn't it dangerous? Won't the wolf get me?' An infant doesn't know that a bed is a safe place, any more than you or I would feel particularly safe in a tent out on the savannah with a pride of lions pawing the tent flaps.

The answer, expressed through your actions, has three aspects and looks something like this:

The Message

The message is given at bedtime. The child is placed on his stomach (the sleep position Hans prefers), the arms are stretched up towards the head of the bed, the legs are straightened, the head is turned towards the right (away from you), and each stage of the process is rounded off with a little pressure.

The room should be cool and dark!

A jingle x 4 is given while you are on the way out, your back turned towards the bed, and is finished outside the door.

The situation is so new (and you are such a new person!) that it may provoke such a strong reaction that you will have to resort to 'buffing'.

You firmly place the child back in position, spread your hand over the little back, apply firm pressure every fourth buff and buff rhythmically with your other hand in a loose fist on the back of the diaper from the bottom up so that the entire little body gets a little nudge every time. This is how to quiet down any baby, no matter how ear-splitting his screams. Hans will quiet down in less than two minutes.

If he doesn't, you will have to perfect your technique (on Mom or your own thighs).

As soon as Hans' body relaxes and he is lying still and breathing regularly, finish off with one last little bit of fanning pressure, which marks the end of the process. Leave the room before *he falls asleep, which sounds as wrong as it is decisively important. The goal is not that you put Hans to sleep – he will only wake up and start to scream because he is not being buffed, which means that you will have to stand by his bed all night! The goal is to enable him to find peace. Hans will go to sleep all by himself, and that means that he will also be able to fall back to sleep all by himself. His sleep becomes his own.*

The Reminder

The reminder is given after carefully monitoring the reaction to the message. Don't be in too much of a hurry. We don't want to impose a prohibition on reacting!

Little Hans is going into the follow-up week now and only needs – in emergencies – a reassuring reminder jingle from the other side of the door (which should be ajar, but not so much that he can see you). The jingle should take over completely during the second night of the cure. But on the first night, the reminder has to be more 'hands on'.

Listen carefully, while the crying or protests – the reaction – either revs up or winds down, which goes in cycles. If you think that the child is really going to rev himself up and get stuck at the top of the wave without being able to wind down again, go back in quickly and quietly and repeat the procedure described above, albeit a shorter and more efficient variant. It should be friendly but firm, as though you are responding to a whiny complaint. 'YES, you can rest easy. NO, the wolf isn't going to get you. There is absolutely NOTHING to worry about! OK, everything is fine now.'

Round off with a little pressure and jingle your way quickly out of the room away from the door without lingering on the threshold. The jingle is the sign off.

From now on, the jingle will constitute the increasingly seldom reminders.

The Confirmation

The confirmation, the last word, is given to merely confirm that all is right with the world. You give it in the form of a confirmation jingle from outside the door. Hans seems to like three rounds. You will feel – 'hear' – that he is receptive. If he isn't receptive right away, if he has had time to get 'stuck' or really wake up, you may have to jingle four times, followed by a fifth jingle, and even a sixth. The jingle should be rhythmically clear, and the final verse should have an obvious ending, very loud if necessary to carry over Hans' voice and get through. It should be friendly but firm. The jingle can also be low and soft if he is quiet, but you still 'hear' that he is wondering whether everything is as it should be, and it can also be given in a slightly angry tone if he is nagging.

By the second night, I was devoting myself exclusively to confirmations – which often began as reminders but segued into concluding confirmations – and I never went back into the room.

Buffing is rewarding and effective but should only be resorted to if it is really necessary! A good rule of thumb for the follow-up week is this: if you feel that going in and buffing is absolutely necessary, that is when you should jingle.

And the jingle should be the same, the words identical. Your goal-oriented jingle will soon evoke a conditioned reflex. Pow! Little Hans will be out like a light.

As you can see, the Good-Night's-Sleep Cure differs dramatically from the so-called Controlled Crying Method or the Five-Minute Method, which have been recommended to you – along with other less than felicitous strategies – by your local children's clinic. Children should not *cry themselves to sleep and be forced to give up, exhausted, despairing and sometimes completely hysterical, with their questions unanswered. They must be given answers immediately.*

Crying for a little while afterwards *is not forbidden* – as long as the cries are not sobs of abandonment, but nothing more than an irritated or angry reaction, which fades into tranquil silence after a minute or two.

Otherwise, a reminder is needed, followed directly by a confirmation, which will be the final word that follows the child into sleep.

That glorious day is approaching, when little Hans knows that he never has to scream out his questions. They will be answered before he even has a chance to think about asking them.

This will be thanks to the schedule, which will make the days and the nights predictable for him. It will also be thanks to his parents, who will ensure that all his needs are met preventively. He will then stop whining and crying. He will hand over responsibility for looking out for his interests to you two. It is an awesome and delightful trust! Which you will not violate by waiting until he really screams before you do something.

It is all about assuming your role as leaders and always being one step ahead of the game. When he is picked up from his bed, it will be at a moment when he is asleep (within the fifteen minute margin) or at least silent and calm. When he is put to bed, he will not be whining from exhaustion but will be as happy as possible, preferably really perky! When he eats and doesn't want any more, he'll have another spoonful if he cries as if he hadn't cried at all, but the meal will end at a moment when he is happy. And so on.

Good times are coming! They will be very, very tired at first. But not for long. And never again.

Eleven and twelve months
The bedtime laugh is a blessing. Happy kids sleep well.

And it doesn't take much to amuse young children – tickling, blowing raspberries on little tummies, making silly faces, hiding behind curtains, pretending to trip, picking up a teddy bear from the floor and exclaiming, 'Look! A hamburger!'

A laugh a day keeps the doctor away and a child free from most problems. Laughing is more than fun. Laughing is essential.

The most important thing for kids around a year old is that their luminous joy isn't clouded.

And nothing kills joy like sleep deprivation. Eleven and twelve-month-old children need between 14 and 13.5 hours sleep a day. And this they will easily get with the help of the *Good-Night's-Sleep Cure*, which has a remarkable effect on them. It liberates the hallmark of every well rested one-year-old: a zest for life.

One-year-olds think that it just rocks to be alive!

And when one sees a little kid this age take on existence with undisguised joy, love and curiosity, one realizes the human species has not survived out of duty or pain or because it is to be pitied.

Life isn't meant to be painful. Life is meant to be joyful and happy. Children around eleven or twelve months old are perhaps the best proof of this.

Therefore – even if this lies a little outside the area of sleep – I will take the opportunity to indulge in a little moral sermon.

- Don't get hung up on the word NO for a good while yet. Give life a free rein!
- Meet your child with a smile! Answer and confirm her zest for life, her unadulterated *joie de vivre!*
- This pure, solid and unhesitating zest for life is ephemeral. Your child's zest for life will never again be as luminously evident as it is now. Share in it!

Every day, young children around a year old give a prim and proper adult the most wonderful opportunity to share that joy, rather than killing it. The way one-year-olds, equipped as they are with four or six teeth, eat an apple for instance injects a little humor into the daily grind!

The apple is acquired and little bits of the skin are gnawed off. These are then spat out. The apple is then deposited somewhere, usually in a corner of the living room, or in the hall, or on top of a book in the book case, or under a radiator.

Two days later the apple is reacquired much to the glee of its owner, who then proceeds to continue eating on the spot. The apple is then placed in a shoe.

When whatever is left of the apple has lain in the shoe for a considerable period of time and collected its share of dirt and dust, turned brown and matured sufficiently, so to speak, its owner has the brilliant idea of giving it to Mom.

Who is absolutely thrilled.

The world is still new, benign and fascinating, even for a one-year-old who has managed to assemble a veritable treasure trove of experience. A dog that appears during a walk is an item of great interest (that can easily become terrifying). A bush with small buds, a branch heavy with snow, a flight of stairs, rough-hewn and inviting, a pavement edge, an old lady with chubby legs, a pile of gravel, a child in a stroller, a bag tossed on the ground...

All this was new to you once too. Once upon a time, you too looked at everything with fresh eyes. Once upon a time, your smile was as glorious and natural as the dawn of a new day. Once upon a time, your laugh was truly your own, born of nothing else but a genuine zest for life.

Cultivate laughter is the evangel of this sermon! Laughter confers a magnificent end to the day and a good sleep – for all concerned.

Little Theo's mother had this to say:
I had wanted to do the Good-Night's-Sleep Cure *for so long, but I kept putting it off because I didn't think we could manage it. Today, my only regret is that we waited so long!*

Our little guy was one when we started the cure. Actually, what I was most nervous about was taking away the pacifier. But it was so easy! The first night, he thought we had gone crazy, but since then he hasn't missed it at all.

Anyway, after much humming and hawing we started the cure, and on the fourth night Theo slept TWELVE hours. We couldn't believe it!

Today, just over a month later, he is still sleeping like a log. He falls asleep effortlessly in the evening and sleeps the whole night, even if he does have a disconcerting habit of waking up a little too early (more often than not because Dad gets up and goes to work). But by and large, everything is working brilliantly! He sleeps, we sleep (yippee!), and the routines are holding up.

When mealtimes roll around, Theo stands at the door to the pantry and bangs on the door until he gets his grub. He is brimming with happiness!

Eleven-month-olds willingly and gratefully accept the sound sleep that the *Good-Night's-Sleep Cure* gives them because they want nothing more than to enjoy that wonderful zest for life that is the hallmark of kids this age.

And as we all know, if this zest for life has a nemesis, it is sleep deprivation.

Little Theo's Mom reiterates:

To all of you out there who are having a hard time with sleepless nights and are thinking about applying the cure, I have only this to say: Don't wait any longer! GO FOR IT! Once you make the decision, it works!

And even if the going gets tough sometimes, you will see the result and this will give you the strength to be both happy and consistent. I'll say it again. GO FOR IT!

Older children

There is no upper age limit for the *Good-Night's-Sleep Cure*. Maybe even thirty-five-year-olds with sleep problems, not to mention pensioners (like me) might derive some benefit from it. However, empirical evidence to support such a proposition is lacking...

The proposition that all children, be they healthy or sick, big or small, both need and *want* to sleep through the night – soundly, peacefully, and sufficiently long – is very easy to support. The *Good-Night's-Sleep Cure*, if applied properly (See *Peace, Security and Enjoyment*) has an obviously liberating effect on children of all ages.

How the strategies and methodology can be adapted to meet the needs of older children will be described in the following chapters. If you took it into your head to try and buff a two-year-old, the kid would at best go into shock and at worst have a seizure... So don't even think about it!

Three and a half years

I have just given our three-and-a-half-year-old the cure.

And just as you said, my daughter thought I was crazy! A girl this 'old' thought that something had just snapped and Mom had taken it into her head that 'Sleep tight. See you in the morning!' was the response to absolutely everything. And my husband agreed with her.

I never buffed. Instead, I held both my hands gently but firmly against her body when she lay down and waited ten seconds before exiting the room with a jingle.

When she spoke loudly, I jingled loudly. When she quieted down, I jingled as softly and delicately as I could.

I got through about forty jingles the first night!

Then she tried to get into our bed three or four times, but I led her back to her room and jingled once I had put her back to bed. The first jingle was firm, but once I had gotten through to her, I softened the tone.

I listened and tried to adjust the jingle to her. And I made sure that I was the one who had the last word and that that last word was tender.

It took two evenings. Then she began to say the jingle to her doll. 'Sleep tight. See you in the morning!' in the cutest tone of voice.

This evening, I simply put her to bed and jingled ONCE. Then I went downstairs and checked out what was on TV.

I only started the cure a week ago. You should also know that she has had problems with going to bed all her life. I can hardly believe how things have changed and I am so relieved! I am stunned by how easy it was to turn the evening and nocturnal torment into its polar opposite!

My daughter is content and secure. She's quite simply a brand new girl. And I'm not just talking evenings and going to bed. I have begun to involve her in everything I do when I get home. She has put a pie together, baked a sponge cake, chopped up salad greens with a (half) sharp knife, wiped the table after dinner and much, much more! All the stuff that I thought she was too young for...

And we always end the day with a laugh.

There was a time when I too thought that peace and quiet was appropriate at bedtime. But she seems to relax if we clown around right up to the time she climbs into bed. I get the feeling that she lies there smiling at all the fun and games, instead of thinking about how horrible it is to sleep alone... She even cracks jokes herself to try and get a laugh out of me when we are sitting on the sofa during our bedtime sessions!

I was desperate before I gave her the Good-Night's-Sleep Cure. *I had tried EVERYTHING (except drugs) with no result. Sometimes our little girl got completely hysterical. She would scream until she threw up and was quite unreachable. She would argue, fight, and be as lippy as you please.*

So I threw myself whole-heartedly into the cure. We had everything to gain and nothing to lose.

Twelve years

I have to tell you something! I have just jingled for my twelve-year-old!

He has been away all weekend visiting a close friend, which obviously means that our routines haven't been followed. I know from experience that the evening after a sleep-over is pretty chaotic, and this evening was no exception. I am usually one step ahead, but this evening I had a bit of a meltdown and wondered desperately what I could do to break the pattern...

He was crying over an autograph that had gone missing and over life generally. He was drinking water straight from the bottle and driving his sister nuts. He was enraged at his uncomprehending mother... I felt insanity creeping up on me.

Then the penny dropped! I began to jingle. 'Good night, sleep tight! See you in the morning!'

'MOM, I'VE GOT BUGS IN MY HAIR!'

'Good night, sleep tight! See you in the morning!'

'I HATE SCHOOL!'

'Good night, sleep tight! See you in the morning!'

And so on.

And do you know what happened? SILENCE! It took five minutes!!!

On an evening like this, he is up and down like a yo-yo, cries and complains, finds a thousand things that he has to get off his chest, and eventually falls into an exhausted sleep at 11 or 12 o'clock, even when we manage to stay calm and firm.

I am so HAPPY! There's hope!

But the best of it is that my son is now calm. He knows that the wolf is being kept at bay and he is sleeping soundly and securely. (Obviously, I'll check his hair in the morning.)

What else is there to say? I think I'll cure my next child while it's still in the womb...!

You fathers and mothers who are wondering whether or not 'jingling' works can stop doubting! If it works on a twelve-year-old, it will work on the President.

III.

THE TOOL BOX. WHEN, WHERE, HOW?

WHEN?

Now we are finally going to get down to business. But I beg you – at the risk of sounding like a nag – read, read, read FIRST!

It is primarily the chapters entitled Peace, Security and Enjoyment that I am referring to.

If and when you decide to apply the *Good-Night's-Sleep Cure*, it is of the utmost importance that you *know exactly what you are doing and why*.

There must be no question marks in your mind at all. Your brain should be choc-a-bloc with *answers* because that is what your child will require of you. It is the child who has exclusive rights to questions here!

When you have ironed out all the kinks and you are so read up on the *Good-Night's-Sleep Cure* that you could teach a course on it for your entire family and half the world, then you are ready to do the job yourself. But first things first!

So I am going to nag a little more – just to be on the safe side.

As you know, we all want our driver's licenses as soon as we decide we want to learn to drive. We want them yesterday. We can't wait to get behind the wheel and simply drive off free as a bird.

But, but, but. There are umpteen things we have to learn first if we don't want the test to go to hell in a hand basket and the license to be gone with the wind.

Whatever we think of the instructor, whatever we think of the manual and whatever we think of the rules of the road, certain things have to be learned if we want to get our hands on that precious license. We can't take shortcuts, cheat, throw out the manual unread, ignore the traffic signs and make up traffic regulations as we go along. We'll just be kicked out of the car and sent back to school.

I know. I *am* nagging... You know all you need to know and then some, right?

Good! You're all set!

• Plan for four days and nights plus a follow-up week. This time must be completely undisturbed. The outside world does not exist.

The *Good-Night's-Sleep Cure* will be eventful enough for all concerned. It requires whole-hearted dedication with as few intrusions as possible.

• You will need a partner in this enterprise. No one can stay awake 24/7.

The first two nights (if you're the one taking them), you can't count on getting any sleep at all.

These nights will be followed by days that must be meticulously organized so that everything hangs together. Your partner must be as read up on his or her subject as you are. (Or at least used to following orders...)

The first couple of days are as important as the first couple of nights. It is now that old patterns of behavior are broken and the new ones must be crystal clear right from the start – if our goal is to make this as easy on the child as possible, which it most certainly is.

Imagine you are teaching a young child to tell the time (which in a way is what you are doing). The prerequisite would be that the hands of the clock function the way they should and the numbers on the clock face stay put. A child wouldn't learn how to tell the time very quickly or very well or at all if the numbers changed places and hands moved at varying speeds. The poor kid would be hopelessly confused.

- It is not uncommon that one of two things happens, once the decision to apply the cure has been taken: 1) the child suddenly starts to sleep like a log or 2) the child gets a terrible cold and her nose runs like a tap. Both will soon pass!

During the *Good-Night's-Sleep Cure* (or even before, as has been seen), it is the child who asks the questions and the cure director (i.e. you) who provides the answers. Thus, you will not place responsibility for starting the cure on the shoulders of your young child but will stick with whatever you have decided.

If your child gets a cold or a fever, he or she *really* needs to sleep at night! Banish any confusion you may be feeling by imagining what you would want – and not want – if *you* were sick.

- The most business-like of the two of you, you brave souls who are going to administer the *Good-Night's-Sleep Cure*, should take care of the first two nights.

It will facilitate things enormously if your cure partner disappears from the family abode and sleeps somewhere else. The first two nights – especially the first – will take their toll. You cannot take care of an anxious/skeptical/ questioning/ protesting/sabotaging adult *too*.

- Once you have taken the capital-D decision, don't surrender even an inch of ground! You are in for the duration. This is no drill.

Don't let anyone or anything stand in your way. These are eleven days and nights that will change your life. If you don't get the support from your surroundings that you would like, remember that it is your *child* who will be the big winner in all this! It is your *child*, who, thanks to you, will receive what is perhaps the greatest gift of all: a sound, secure, pleasurable sleep.

Sound sleep is a gift that lasts a lifetime! (And when those around see how blissfully your child sleeps, you will be told how 'lucky' you are to have such a 'good' baby...)

The support that you don't get from the people around you will be made up for by the support you receive from your child, once all the puzzle pieces fall into place.

And rewards don't get any better than that.

WHERE?

The young child who is to be cured needs her own separate sleeping space. No visual input must be allowed to penetrate.

Ninety percent of a young child's sensory input is visual, and if there is something to look at, that little brain immediately cranks into gear. During the night, when the goal is a sound, continuous, long sleep, we don't want any visual input at all. It's disturbing. (Hearing 'All is well', or a variation thereof, is not disturbing at all however – quite the contrary!)

Invest in a crib! It serves as a miniature room for children between the ages of four months and at least three years. It's a blessing, I think (and children think so too). Think about where it can be permanently placed.

• In a separate room?

Then blackout curtains must be placed over the windows so that not even a glimmer of light can find its way in. No light from the hall must fall on the child either, whether the door is merely ajar or wide open.

• In a corner in the parents' bedroom?

The corner should be deep enough to screen off with blackout curtains from floor to ceiling (although air must be able to circulate). A ceiling rod is not that hard to put up. Leave enough room between the bed and the curtains so that the little angel can't open them herself and peek out!

You and your partner must also resign yourselves to the fact that you will *not* be able to sleep in your bedroom for the first four nights, during which the child must not be exposed to the presence of others. It's about respect. And, yes, I know that loving parents don't want to believe that their presence could ever disturb their adored child, but, alas, it does at night. (See *Security.*)

During the follow-up week, you can sneak in to sleep, but until the nights have 'settled' properly, you must be prepared to pretend that you don't really exist. And be sure to sneak soundlessly out the room before you jingle from outside the door.

- Can a corner in the living room perhaps serve as the child's room if you live in cramped quarters?

Space can always be found if you put your mind to it. You may even be able to clear a spot in the living room that really can function as a little 'room' with space for a bureau, shelves and various other accoutrements.

An angled rod in the ceiling can work miracles. Blackout curtains that allow air to circulate are available by the square yard in every conceivable color.

And you should understand that life in the living room can go on as per normal as soon as you have reached the final goal – enjoyment – and your child has become a Sound Sleeper!

A little eight-month-old boy, whom I cured in a single night when he was four months (the parents then took over), got a makeshift 'room' in the living room, where the noise level was sometimes so extreme that the neighbors complained. The parents were very young. They had an army of friends who liked nothing better than to hang out in the parents' apartment in the evening to watch TV, dance to disco music, talk, laugh, eat and drink and sing Karaoke.

More often than not, they did all this at once...

And the baby slept.

Finally, one of the girls, who doubted that there was really a baby behind the curtains, felt compelled to check for herself. How could a baby sleep through all that racket? She looked through the curtains. And let in some light.

The baby awoke with a start, groped his way up into a sitting position and began to cry heartrendingly.

For a long time, that little boy was inconsolable. Someone had invaded his room! His security hung in the balance! Someone had *disturbed* him!

• The room should be cool. Preferably cold. Can you arrange that?

Children who sleep in a really cool room don't kick their covers off (except at the beginning of the cure when they don't lie still). You can dispense with all the sleep overalls, sleeping bags and thick pajamas! What young children invariably love best is *freedom of movement*. Arms and legs would not be imprisoned in warm clothes at night if young children had anything to say about it. A little body suit or a roomy T-shirt that covers the diaper is ideal.

• Make the bed with a soft bottom sheet and tuck it in firmly so that everything is tight and smooth. A terry towel under the bottom sheet is a good idea.

A little four-month-old may need a couple of tightly rolled baby blankets on each side so she can 'burrow' down a little.

Tummy sleepers appreciate a sheet folded in three and tucked in around the mattress at the head of the bed. This folded sheet will add a little height and will stay smooth and in position when the baby turns her head during the night.

Back sleepers need a small down pillow, which should be flat and soft. This pillow should be more soft than flat, since we want to avoid so-called 'flat skull' (which will not return to normal after six months).

The quilt or fairly thick blanket that goes on top should be soft, clean and easy to wash. *One* little stuffed animal is permitted, but no more than that.

Remember that it can be a bit stressful for the baby to keep track of too many accessories in the dark. So, be frugal!

The pacifier, that true disturber of the peace, will disappear on the first evening. The child will forget all about it that very night. You might not think that is possible, but seeing is believing!

• Buy an apnea alarm and put it in the bed!

So called breathing alarms are no longer restricted to hospitals but are available to the general public, and that is a blessing.

Place the sensor plate under the mattress, which will not disturb the child in the least, but will do wonders for your own nerves. A small light blinks reassuringly on the accompanying monitor, which can be placed somewhere prominent. You will be spared all that anxiety over your child's breathing, which is impossible to check on every three minutes. Since the alarm works on the same principle as the smoke detector you have hopefully installed in your home, it will monitor your child's breathing pattern around the clock.

The smoke detector doesn't guarantee that your house won't catch fire, any more than the breathing monitor guarantees that your child won't stop breathing, but you will have ample warning. You will have time to prevent the catastrophe that *could* have happened. You have nothing to lose and everything to gain.

Breathing is not automatic at the beginning of life – newborns stop breathing for as long as forty seconds several times a day, something that few adults could manage.

Since I would rather be safe than sorry, I would maintain that you should operate under the assumption that breathing is not guaranteed until your child is ten to eleven months old.

- Nothing prevents you from seeing through the first few days and nights of the cure outside your home.

You shouldn't have to worry about what the neighbors will think (and there *will* be a good deal of crying, questioning and protesting, especially during the first night. It is unavoidable unless we gag the child. And that is something we definitely don't want to do. We want to communicate!).

Nor is there anything that prevents someone other than yourself or the child's other parent from administering the cure. I am walking proof. Even though I was a complete stranger, I cured hundreds of children in my home, a totally unfamiliar environment.

The important thing is that *one and the same person* takes care of the first two nights, and then adequately prepares whoever takes charge of the following two.

The days that follow the first two nights should also be looked after by the same person – although obviously not the person who looks after the nights. (The cure begins in the evening.) It is then that a carefully planned schedule is introduced. This schedule must be followed to the letter, which is not easy at the beginning since the child is completely confused.

However, as early as the third day, several puzzle pieces fall into place and the child begins to set her own little internal clock.

The cure directors should still be two, and the same two, wherever the child happens to be, and the place should be the same for at least three of the first four days and nights.

When you eventually get home, everything should have been prepared as outlined above so that you can continue the cure in peace and quiet.

A father's story follows:
It seems like an eternity since we cured Felix. Still, it's only been a few months...

We were so exhausted both mentally and physically that if I hadn't found Anna's forum, I don't know what would have become of us.

We thought that the status quo was completely normal, and we were just wait-

ing for everything to somehow blow over. Every evening we were optimistic. *This night is going to be better...* This worked for the first year, but by the second year we were running on empty.

Unfortunately, a lot of people think it is completely normal that children don't sleep until they turn two! It's just a fact of life, so suck it up and get over it. What lunacy!

I fell into that trap too, even though I had trouble understanding why it had to be that way. I listened to the people with expertise and experience (yeah right!). The whole thing makes me shiver now, especially when I think about all those poor little kids, who are the ones who suffer the most. Sleep deprivation is just their lot in life for the first couple of years. How insanely illogical is that? If ever you should be able to sleep without a care in the world, it is then, all the while secure in the knowledge that your parents are looking after you.

The first time I tried the cure, I didn't have the will power to see it through. When I fanned the boy, I couldn't take the sobs that came with all the questions. It was a half-hearted attempt that was doomed to failure. But I read about other people's attempts on the forum, and that gave my motivation a shot in the arm. Those who succeeded wrote that it was actually very simple as long as you kept your eye on the prize and didn't give up.

I began to think about trying again, but I wanted to be properly prepared this time.

It took a few months, but finally I thought it was time. I slept during the day so that I could stay awake the first night. I felt confident, but a little nervous nonetheless.

We had agreed that Mom would sleep in another room, so she wouldn't have to get involved in what I was doing. She said that she couldn't handle it.

Of course it felt a little strange to force the child into a prone position, especially since he was already so big. But decisive is as decisive does. And it couldn't be worse than letting him wake up so many times or simply leaving him to scream. I was, after all, close to him and even had physical contact with him.

I remember reading a piece on the forum where the parents described how they had decided not to proceed because they thought that fanning was tantamount to physical abuse... But isn't it even more abusive to let the child cry for a couple of years?

Already on the first night, falling asleep was easier. I remember that I was so chuffed that, with the fanning, it took exactly 45 minutes, just as Anna had said.

I no longer remember how many times he woke up those first nights, but it wasn't that many nights before he was sleeping his twelve continuous hours. We couldn't believe it! We had such trouble wrapping our minds around it that we didn't know how to react. It felt like magic...

The daytime naps were just as smooth. It was just a matter of putting him down, and presto! he was asleep. Just like that, no muss no fuss. And he was happy as a clam too. That was plain to see. So were we of course. It was so wonderful to know that he was sleeping through the night without any problems. We could sleep too at long last... It took a few months before we were back up to par, but we made it. Now we enjoy our child in a completely different way! Both child and parents have the strength to do so much more.

Felix is still sleeping through the night. Sometimes he wakes up a little too early, but it's nothing I worry about, since, come what may, he sleeps the entire night without waking up.

The strange thing is that it feels like a luxury when in fact it is completely normal!

To any of you out there who read this and still hesitate, I just want to say that the fact that your child isn't sleeping through the night is something that can be changed. Most parents think that their own child is so special that this cure won't work. I also thought that my child was too old, along with a host of other misgivings. I'd made sure that every imaginable escape hatch was open.

All the information that has to be mastered can be a little frightening too.

But in the end, it was so simple that I was almost mad at myself because I hadn't done something sooner. If you have come this far, you are already halfway to the finish line. All you have to do is study the material, prepare yourself and pick the night that will change your lives...

Father to Felix, born March 2005, cured January 2007.

HOW? THE TOOL BOX

- The Schedule
- The Bedtime Laugh
- Corrective Positioning
- Fanning
- Rocking
- Buffing
- The Good Night Jingle
- The Confirmation Jingle
- An Attitude of Supreme Confidence

The Schedule

Do your thinking with a pencil and paper. First, decide when the night is going to begin so that it fits in with family life.

And how long is the night to be? Twelve hours, eleven or eleven and a half?

Continue with meal planning. You're aiming for four substantial meals a day with three to three and a half hours in between, as well as an evening top up just before bedtime.

The evening top up is the exception that proves the rule; it can be given as little as an hour after 'dinner'.

Then move on to the daytime naps. In *Children and Sleep*, the sleep requirements per every 24-hour period were specified for the various age groups. Here you will need to do a little math. If, for example, you choose an 11.5 hour night for your seven to eight month-old little angel, that leaves three hours out of a total requirement of 14.5 hours that has to be spread over three daytime naps.

Five minutes, 20 minutes, 45 minutes, 1.5 hours, 2 hours and 3 hours are nap durations that best suit a child's natural sleep rhythms. Once these time periods have elapsed, children drift up towards consciousness and are easily awoken.

Plan this carefully! The schedule must be so well thought out that you wouldn't even dream of adjusting it until the follow-up week is over and done with, at the earliest. Once it has been 'signed and sealed', it must not be questioned!

Here are some examples of how the schedule might look:

Philip, *four months.* Total sleep requirement 15.5/24
Night 8.00 p.m. to 7.00 a.m.
Feeding 7.00 a.m.
Nap 8.30 a.m. to 10.00 a.m. (1.5 hours)
Feeding 10.00 a.m.
Nap 11.30 a.m. to 1.00 p.m. (1.5 hours)
Feeding 1.00 p.m.
Nap 3.00 p.m. to 3.45 p.m. (45 minutes)
Feeding 4.00 p.m.
Nap 5.45 p.m. to 6.30 p.m. (45 minutes)
Top up 7.30 p.m.
Down for the night 8.00 p.m.

The meals – which should not last more than an hour at most (in another month little Philip will be down to a maximum of 45 minutes) – are spliced in so that they are consistently three hours apart.

This, together with the fact that the night is eleven hours long and not twelve, means that it's a bit of a long haul until the evening top up. Consequently, the top up should be supplemented with something appropriate over and above breast milk if the child is still being breastfed.

These are the kinds of things that have to be mulled over when you are making up a schedule!

Emma, *five months.* Total sleep: 15 hours 15 minutes/24
Night 8.00 p.m. to 7.00 a.m.
Feeding 7.00 a.m.
Nap 8.00 a.m. to 8.45 a.m. (45 minutes)

Feeding 8.45 a.m.
Nap 9.45 a.m. to 10.30 a.m. (45 minutes)
Feeding 12.00 noon
Nap 1.00 p.m. to 3.00 p.m. (2 hours)
Feeding 3.00 p.m.
Nap 5.00 p.m. to 5.45 p.m. (45 minutes)
Feeding/Top up 6.30 p.m.
Down for the night 8.00 p.m.

There are several things to contemplate here, as you can see. The first nap is spliced in only an hour after the night ends, and the second meal is given sooner than the stipulated three hours. There is only an hour and 45 minutes between meal one and meal two.

The reason is simple. All her young life, little Emma has shown herself to be so groggy in the mornings that her father and I had to take that into account when we put her schedule together (see page 110). The second meal turned into a second breakfast.

One month later, when Emma was *six months*, the schedule was adjusted because she had gotten older. Then Dad shortened the afternoon nap to 20 minutes.

The next month, when little Emma was *seven months* old, the family let the afternoon nap fall by the wayside and the night began at 7.00 p.m. Thus, Emma got her twelve hours of night sleep.

The long nap at midday or in the early afternoon can be retained for several years, so take this into account from the start!

During the first year, the order in which these naps are dispensed with is as follows: the afternoon nap goes first, the second morning nap (if there is one) second, and the first morning nap last.

Oliver, *seven months*. Total sleep: 14 hours 35 minutes/24
Night 8.30 p.m. to 8.30 a.m.
Feeding 8.30 a.m.

Nap 10.30 a.m. to 11.15 a.m. (45 minutes)
Feeding 12.00 noon
Nap 1.30 p.m. to 3.00 p.m. (1.5 hours)
Feeding 3.00 p.m.
Nap 5.15 p.m. to 5.35 p.m. (20 minutes)
Feeding 7.00 p.m.
Bath, fun and games, top up 7.30 p.m. to 8.30 p.m.
Down for the night 8.30 p.m.

Plan to set aside one hour in the evening for all the fun and games that should precede the short bedding procedure!

A bath is a wonderful end to the day and will soon be associated with a good night's sleep.

Laura, *eight months*. Total sleep: 14 hours 35 minutes /24
Night 7.30 p.m. to 7.30 a.m.
Feeding 7.30 a.m.
Nap 10.00 a.m. to 10.45 a.m. (45 minutes)
Feeding 11.00 a.m.
Nap 12.30 p.m. to 2.00 p.m. (1.5 hours)
Feeding 2.00 p.m.
Nap 4.00 p.m. to 4.20 p.m. (20 minutes)
Feeding 4.45 p.m.
Bath, fun and games, top up 6.30 p.m. to 7.30 p.m.
Down for the night 7.30 p.m.

Little Laura will soon turn **nine months**, and her sleep requirement will diminish by half an hour.

She will announce this by suddenly starting to wake up way too early in the mornings. She may also indicate that times they are a-changing by questioning the one-and-a-half-hour midday nap. This she will do by waking up after forty-five minutes and not going back to sleep. Young children 'tell' their caregivers when it's time to revise the schedule.

And since Laura's loving parents know that everything is interlocked, they will not shorten the night. The twelve hour night will stay in force for several years. If Laura calls the afternoon nap into question, they will pay no attention. It stays as is.

Instead, they will shorten the morning nap from 45 minutes to 20, which will tick Laura off no end for the first few days. After all, she never woke up too early from *that* nap.

But in three or four days, she adjusts to the new order, and thereafter does not wake up too early in the mornings.

Terry, *nine months*. Total sleep requirement: 14 hours 15 minutes
Night 7.00 p.m. to 7.00 a.m.
Feeding 7.00 a.m.
Morning games in bed 7.15 a.m. to 8.15 a.m.
Feeding (second breakfast) 8.15 a.m.
Nap 9.15 a.m. to 10.00 a.m. (45 minutes)
Feeding 11.30 a.m.
Nap 12.30 p.m. to 2.00 p.m. (1.5 hours)
Feeding 3.00 p.m.
Feeding (dinner with the family) 5.30 p.m.
Bath, fun and games, top up 6.00 p.m. to 7.00 p.m.
Down for the night 7.00 p.m.

Terry has six meals spliced into his schedule. This particular piece of planning has a social dimension. He partakes of a 'real' breakfast and a 'real' dinner with the family every day. His own meals satisfy the caloric requirements for a young child his age. At the table with his parents, he can scope out what *they* eat and acquaint himself with something called 'gastronomic culture'.

Amanda, *ten months*. Total sleep: 14 hours 15 minutes
Night 7.00 p.m. to 7.00 a.m.

Feeding 7.00 a.m.
Nap 8.45 a.m. to 9.30 a.m. (45 minutes)
Feeding 10.30 a.m.
Nap 12.00 noon to 1.30 p.m. (1.5 hours)
Feeding 2.00 p.m.
Feeding 5.30 p.m.
Bath, fun and games, top up 6.00 p.m. to 7.00 p.m.
Down for the night 7.00 p.m.

Little Amanda always finishes eating within half an hour. The meals are consistently spaced three and a half hours apart. The top up before bed is the exception.

With a twelve-hour night behind her, Amanda manages just fine on only two naps a day.

Orson, *one year.* Total sleep requirement: 13 hours 30 minutes
Night 8.00 p.m. to 7.30 a.m.
Feeding (oatmeal porridge with mashed banana and milk + a sandwich) 8.00 a.m.
Outdoor play and social participation
Feeding (lunch with 'real' food) 11.30 a.m.
Midday nap 12.30 p.m. to 2.30 p.m. (2 hours)
Feeding (snack: fruit and yoghurt, or sandwich with milk) 3.00 p.m.
Outdoor play and social participation
Feeding (dinner with parents) 6.30 p.m.
Bath, fun and games, top up 7.00 p.m. to 8.00 p.m.
Down for the night 8.00 p.m.

Little Orson's parents are home free, you might say. His schedule will not need adjusting for several years.

Preferably, the schedule you devise should be followed to the letter during the first four days and nights of the cure! During the follow up week and thereafter, you can allow yourself a fifteen minute margin in either direction.

And the times must stay the same, day and night, weekdays and weekends. I can understand how you might think it all sounds a little boring, but it isn't! To go back to the driver's license analogy, you would hardly *begin* your career as driver by calling into question all the rules of the road and only obeying road signs when you felt like it.

So think the schedule through very carefully and then stick to it come hell or high water. Make your watch your best friend.

Before your child becomes her own clock, you will have to wake her occasionally if you are to stick to the schedule. Naturally, this goes against the grain, now that she is finally sleeping blissfully. But don't be afraid to take charge. That is precisely what your child expects of you (and she has been waiting a long time). You can take heart from the fact that, at long last, *you know exactly what you are doing and why.*

The Bedtime Laugh

When was the last time you had a good laugh? Is it really possible to laugh too much? I certainly don't think so!

The importance of laughter is underestimated in our culture. A good laugh promotes good health.

Your child should have at least one good laugh a day, preferably in the evening. Ideally, a child should laugh all the way to bed! You can pretend you are an airplane and fly her to the bedroom. You can dance your way to bed with the child on your head... It won't take you long to dream up something unbeatable!

It is not always easy to get a laugh out of an overtired child, so you will have to make an effort. Anything goes, as long as you manage to elicit a loud, hearty laugh (even if it is somewhat reluctant in the beginning). Don't hesitate to tickle her if that's what it takes! Laughter is obligatory!

The Bedtime Laugh should not only be heard. Your child should feel it throughout her entire body. The Bedtime Laugh is *de rigeur!*

Corrective Positioning

Corrective positioning sends a signal to a young child's brain that all activity must cease.

Instead of carefully laying the child down and hoping for the best, while you silently bombard the child with anxious questions and pleas ('Please sleep for a while. It would be so good for all of us!'), you are taking charge with a firm grip, a decisive attitude and gentle but confident power.

Practice corrective positioning on your partner when he or she is in a frisky mood! When you get to the stage of correctively positioning a child, you must know exactly what you are doing and why. The whole point is that you know your stuff.

For *young children* – tummy sleepers and back sleepers – there are three distinct steps:

- Arms up
- Legs stretched out
- Head to the right (away from you)

The little arms should be laid up around the head. Apply light pressure when they are in position so that they 'land'.

Stretch out both legs simultaneously, your hands around the little knee caps and let them land too with a little pressure once they are in place.

Finally, take the head between your palms, turn it away from you and set it down on its side with light pressure. Ideally, your child will not be able to see anything with her head so positioned.

Now contact between the two of you is broken, and you leave the child to her sleep, which is hers and hers alone.

Naturally, the little angel will immediately pull her arms down and her legs up, and that is permitted. The main thing is that you unequivocally 'park' the child so that the message gets through. *All activity will now cease.*

As soon as the initial confusion dissipates – during the second 24 hours of the cure – your child will park herself just fine with only a little help from you. You pull up the arms and presto! the child stretches out her own legs. Message received and understood!

Older children of more than a year (who cannot be either 'rocked' or 'buffed') are placed in their favorite position, which is usually on their sides. Corrective positioning is applied to the position, so to speak.

Pressure is applied in the same order: arms first, legs second, head last.

If the head is turned towards you, corrective positioning is best applied in the dark.

To conclude the procedure, apply fanning pressure over the whole body for a few seconds (see below).

Fanning

Spread your hands as wide as you can and hold them in front of you so that you have a double fan. You are going to place both your hands on the child so that you cover as much of the little body as possible.

You are then going to apply gentle but firm static pressure. Use two of your outer finger tips to keep the head in place.

Fanning involves applying vertical pressure. You are confirming the corrective positioning physically. Now it's time to lie still. (See *Peace.*)

This technique is used for emphasis after corrective positioning and buffing (see below).

Young Children

Fanning works best of course if the child is lying on her stomach, since the 'shell' protects the delicate parts. (Imagine a little turtle!) But even if the child is lying on her side, it sends a distinctly tranquilizing message.

If your child is absolutely determined to lie on her back, be careful not to apply pressure on these delicate parts (the abdomen, upper rib cage and throat).

Older Children

'Fanning' a disoriented, tense kid who thinks that *you* are the wolf is hardly a walk in the park. You have read the report from Felix's dad above. He devoted a grand total of 45 minutes to fanning his son before the message went home in a way that satisfied both parties.

In cases such as this, fanning is the only tool available (apart from the jingle afterwards of course), since the child is too big for buffing. I would argue that even people old enough to be drawing pensions can be fanned...

If you are using fanning to send a message – *now it's time to lie still* – you are looking at a time frame of five to ten seconds.

If fanning is employed to defuse a crisis, you will have to play it by ear. It will take as long as it takes. It has to be forceful enough to prevent the child from twisting and turning her head or her body.

As I'm sure you understand, fanning will not win you any popularity contests the first time you use it. No human being, big or small, likes being restrained. It takes time for a child to allow herself to feel that she is in fact fairly comfortable and indeed rather tired – very tired.

The child's little body must be heavy with sleep before you take the pressure off and stop fanning (with one final brief application), so take your time. Better too much than too little.

In a crisis situation, it doesn't matter if the child has had time to fall asleep by the time you are finished. The jingle (see below) will follow you out of the room in any case, thus giving you the last word. It will enter the child's consciousness 'through the back door'.

If you feel you are being violent and cruel by holding your child in position and implacably resisting her frantic efforts to break free, consider two things:

- If you are using fanning to defuse a crisis for the first time, rest assured it will never again take as long for your reassuring message to get through (as long as you don't abandon the fight before the goal of a sleep heavy little body is reached).

152

- The force, the 'violence' you use, is no worse than the violence you will be forced to resort to if and when your child refuses to allow herself to be strapped into her car seat.

    There are certain things that are simply not negotiable. Life is what it is.

Rocking

The first order of business is to get yourself a good baby carriage. It should be roomy and have a flat bottom (for tummy sleepers).

Young children who have taken a shine to sleeping on their stomachs prefer this position during daytime naps too, so investing in an ancient, second hand extra carriage is a good idea.

A second carriage can also be for exclusive use indoors.

But little back sleepers like being rocked too, and there are many young children who sleep on their stomachs at night and on their backs during daytime naps – although for shorter periods. Tummy sleepers have an advantage in that they can change position and move more easily than the 'locked' back sleepers, who tend to wake up after 20 or 45 minutes and seldom sleep continuously during a long nap of 1.5 or two hours (or even three if that is what you have decided on).

The carriage should be roomy enough for a little tummy sleeper to move her arms down to her side easily after they have been positioned upwards. There should also be sufficient room for the child to extend her legs fully.

When you are planning your child's night sleep and naps, you should be *consistent.*

During the *Good-Night's-Sleep Cure's* first four days and nights, as well as during the follow-up week, everything should be as predictable as possible. The child can sleep in the carriage during the day and the bed at night, she can take one nap in the carriage indoors and the other outdoors, she can sleep in the crib both at night and during the midday nap, or any other combination you choose, but bear in mind that the days (and the nights) should be identical.

Crisp, preferably very cool air promotes good sleep, and provided your child is properly covered, she can take all naps outdoors during the day (unless the weather conditions are extreme).

N.B. The apnea alarm can go off if the carriage is moving. It can even be set off by the wind. You will have to stop the carriage often and check the breathing. And don't forget to turn the alarm on as soon as you stop the carriage for a stationary nap.

Effective rocking is an art. Place something in the carriage that corresponds to your child's weight and take the time to perfect your talents before you begin the cure.

- Make sure you have lots of room. Push the weighted carriage away from you and fully extend your arm.
- Pull it back with a powerful jerk – imagine the carriage was about to roll down a hill and you managed to catch it just in time.
- Push the carriage away from you again, also with a powerful jerk. (I usually bounce the carriage off my hip.)
- Repeat and get a rhythm going. One-two-buckle-your-shoe, three-four-shut-the-door. Fully extend your arm every time and then some. You will understand what I am getting at once you try it!

The goal of rocking is *peace*, not comfort or sleep. So you have to put your back into it. You are sending a *message*, not asking a host of insecure questions (or questions of any description). This is not about mutual communication. To put it brutally, the goal is to *shock* the child into silence!

Thus, this is not a matter of careful, delicate little movements of the carriage. Such movements are reserved for peaceful walks. This kind of delicate rocking is something all young children adore and it will put them to sleep beautifully, back sleepers included. However, delicate rocking will not work if the goal is to cure a baby with sleep problems. Only robust rocking will do!

If you revert to delicate rocking and soothing, two things will inevitably happen: 1) the child will sense danger the minute the carriage stops moving, and she will wake up and cry, and 2) you will find yourself stuck in the much talked about 'rocking trap' and you will have to rock the entire night/nap.

When you start practicing, imagine that the howling baby in carriage must be silenced in a fraction of a second. You grapple with carriage as though it were about to go over a cliff. You won't get a second chance so you had better make sure your grip is secure. If you have a firm grip on the carriage, you will have a firm handle on the situation!

Effective rocking will calm even a hysterically screaming child in less than two minutes.

Practice two minute sessions. End with a series of rapid movements of the handle from side to side for about as long as it takes you to count to five. Then immediately turn away from the carriage and *leave*, taking the wolves of anxiety with you.

After a break that exceeds two minutes, *longer* than the time you spent rocking, go back for a new session and work on your technique. Continue until you have gotten the hang of the jerk (in both directions) and found the right rhythm and pace. When you have a child instead of a weight in the carriage, you will not only understand *how* effective rocking works but also *that* it works!

The opposite of security is insecurity, and insecurity must be banished from rocking and from child care in general. Insecurity will lead you straight to the rocking trap and, even worse, provides you with no tools to give your child *security*. That is why it is so important to work on your rocking technique.

Once you have gotten the jerk, the pace and the rhythm down pat, imagine that you have a little baby (a tummy sleeper we will assume) who stubbornly persists in lifting up her head, thereby reducing her chances of finding the peace she needs. Or perhaps she keeps on raising her whole upper body. Use your free hand to make half a fan, and every time your draw the carriage towards you (or push it away from you, whichever works best), give the head and upper body a fleeting but decisive push downwards.

You can also use this technique to signal that corrective positioning remains in force, regardless of whether or not the child is making any attempt to 'raise' herself.

As previously stated, effective rocking is an art... But don't despair! If I can learn to do it, so can you, and so can everyone else.

And when you have courageously mastered this art, you will soon have to put it back in the Tool Box. Life isn't fair, is it?!

Like buffing, rocking is a tool for conveying *a message that induces peace*, rather than a message that soothes or comforts. This peace inducing message does not have to be conveyed very often (see *Peace*), provided you convey it in a way the child finds convincing.

And this you will do, since it is the *child* that needs this peace.

As early as the second 24 hours of the *Good-Night's-Sleep Cure*, when the child has begun to accept the message that there are no wolves on the horizon (and the darkness is nothing to be afraid of either), you can let the jingle take up more and more of the slack. And your child, who has already learned to appreciate rocking (so horrid at first), just as kids who have been buffed to peace learn to appreciate buffing (so horrid at first), will start to protest over *that* in the form of persistent nagging. You will hear all about it!

Then it is a question of extricating yourself from the rocking trap and the buffing trap and answering with the jingle instead. And make sure that the confirmation jingle is the last word.

This is how you work in *security*. (See the chapter with the same title.) This security is something the child will carry within herself and for herself, just as her sleep is hers and hers alone.

The transition consists of three stages:

- Corrective positioning, rocking, jerking the handle of the carriage, jingle
- Corrective positioning, jerking the handle of the carriage, jingle
- Corrective positioning, jingle.

Buffing

Buffing can be compared to rocking and is based on the same principle: The little body will be helped to peace with the same back-and-forth movements that energetic rocking involves. The difference is that it is you and your buffing movements, rather than those of the carriage, which induce peace so efficiently.

It is perfectly possible, as you understand, to buff even a very young child to peace.

Once you have decided to administer the *Good-Night's-Sleep Cure* to a little baby who is suffering from sleep problems, meticulous training is required before you start to buff. Begin by practicing on your own thighs.

- Sit with your legs slightly apart. Imagine that the right thigh is the baby's diapered bottom and the left thigh is the baby's back, shoulders and neck.
- Make a loose fist with your right hand and turn your hand upwards and towards you so that you can see all your fingernails. Your thumb is pointing away from you and the outer side of your hand is turned towards the thigh that is doubling as your child's diapered bottom.
- Make a broad fan with your left hand over your left thigh, which is where your child's back would be. Place your hand on your thigh and apply light pressure.
- Begin to buff against your right thigh with the outer side of your loosely clenched right fist and your wrist. Count out loud: one, two, three, four. Your up turned hand will help you control the direction from the relaxed mobile wrist joint.
- Increase the pressure slightly. Your thigh should move noticeably with each buff. The pressure you apply while you are buffing is gentle and empathetic, but firm and decisive. But there is nothing harsh about it. You are not hitting or hurting yourself. You are just 'nudging', but it is distinctly felt. You should be able to tap your foot to the beat!
- With your fanned out left hand, hold your left thigh in place so that it is not knocked out of position when your right thigh is buffed against

it. Now apply a little more pressure with your fanned out hand with every fourth buff and then reduce the pressure again. Buff, count, apply pressure. ONE, two, three four... ONE, two, three, four. Rhythm and pace is required. Do this to music if it helps. ONE, two, three four... ONE, two, three, four!

- Round it all off by applying gentle but firm pressure with both hands spread into fans over both thighs, which represent the child's whole body.

When you feel you have the routine down, you can graduate from your thighs to your cure partner! And he or she can practice on you.

- Get your partner into the appropriate position on the sofa: arms up, legs out, head to the right and away from you. (Having fun is not forbidden.) Your partner can play the role of contrary infant so that you learn to set things right without being unpleasant. Friendly but firm is your motto!
- Spread your left hand into a fan, as wide as you can, and hold your partner's head in place with a finger tip or two with the rest of your fingers pressing on part of your partner's back.
- Start buffing. You are now working with your loosely clenched right fist directly aimed at the precious target. Your wrist is relaxed and you are making firm nudging movements. Your partner has no diaper so you are working on his or her buttock.
- Imagine you are pushing in a certain direction, a nudge to your partner's whole body every time you buff, while at the same time you are resisting by keeping your left hand in position and applying pressure.
- Count to yourself: one, two, three, four (pressure to the back), ONE, two, three, four... Find the rhythm!
- Buffing should be perceived as calming and reassuring, friendly but decisive, and essentially peace inducing. Your partner should grade you on this! Your movements must not irritate or upset, and there must not be anything clumsy or uncertain about them. And of course, your buffing should not hurt, no matter how firm you have to be. Your partner should be able to relax and *want* to relax thanks to your rhythmic ministrations.

- Change places when your partner is satisfied (hopefully he or she will want you to continue). 'This is better than Shiatsu and it's free!' Your partner can then practice on you. You will then experience what your child does. You will know how it feels, what you like and what you don't like, and by extension, what your child likes and doesn't like. You will have a handle on what feels so relaxing that it sends you off to sleep!

Buffing, like fanning, is applied vertically so that direction and pressure can be controlled. Your back won't appreciate your having to stand bent over, especially during the first marathon buffing session that can take between 20 and 45 minutes. But you can comfort yourself with the thought this is a one off. *It will never take this long again.*

For a young child with sleep problems, the bed is swarming with wolves. Your child has feared the wolf right from the beginning, and with good reason, but it was not your child who invited the wolf to take up permanent residence in the bed. It was you... (See *Security*). You are being punished for your sins! Look at things from the other side of the fence and try to cheer yourself up (and your back) with the prospect of a wolf-free bed in only 20 to 45 minutes!

The next time your child wakes up, you will only have to buff for a couple of minutes (same drill as with rocking).

And during the second night of the *Good-Night's-Sleep Cure*, it's time to put buffing back in the Tool Box. At this point, the jingle takes over.

N.B. Young children who have been buffed to peace in a roomy crib and jingled, and who have fallen asleep by themselves for the first time love dozing off in just about every conceivable position: lying diagonally on top of the covers, curled up in a ball at the foot of the crib, bent double or even sitting up. Lying with one leg (or both) sticking out through the railings of the crib is another option. (Just be aware that the sides of the crib should have safety guards if your child is younger than six months.)

Resist the temptation to check on your child until you are sure she has been asleep for ten minutes (not 20)! Then go in quickly and adjust the covers. You can even lift the child and position her in the bed without disturbing her.

When you are done, make your exit quietly and discreetly! (If your child does take it into her head to pose a question, answer with a confirmation jingle from outside the door.)

As you have no doubt noticed, I am a shameless advocate of putting babies to bed on their stomachs. (Yes, I can imagine your terrified objections. The following statistic may allay your worst fears. To this day there is not one documented case of SIDS anywhere in the world of the deceased baby having slept in the prone position while equipped with an onset breathing alarm.)

I don't advocate this solely because I think that it is so much simpler and more efficient to both rock and buff a child who is lying on her stomach, not to mention how much it facilitates corrective positioning and fanning. I also champion this cause because the prone position in and of itself is sleep inducing for infants.

The fact is that young children who sleep on their stomachs from day one seldom develop sleep problems.

'Frog sleeping' is as natural for a human child as it is for all other life forms with four limbs, none of whom willingly go to sleep with their vital organs exposed and their legs in the air.

A newborn baby can lift her head, turn it from side to side and take in air. Lying on her stomach, an infant has a freedom of movement that is compromised if she is placed on her back.

Changing position is something we all need to do, even when we are asleep – if we can.

The advantages of tummy sleeping are incontestable. Here are a few of them:

- That little digestive system, which is still developing, has a much easier ride if its owner sleeps on her stomach.
- Runny noses drain.
- Burps and spit ups can't cause catastrophes.
- The risk of suffocation is eliminated if the bottom of the crib is smooth.

If something happens to be covering the back of the baby's skull, all she has to do is lift her head.

- Infants who lie on their stomachs can practice those *neurologically essential crawling movements* from day one, which aids in the healthy development of motor skills and all five senses.

Sophia's mother tells her story:
By and large, Sophia slept terribly right from the start and things went from bad to worse. She would wake up once an hour all night. I would carry her around in my arms from dusk to dawn, but that made things worse rather than better. Then, when she was four and a half months old, I decided to go for the cure. We just didn't have the strength to get through the nights anymore.

It went very well, in spite of one temporary derailment, and Sophia now sleeps fine at night. She used to have a poor appetite, but only a couple of days of the cure fixed that.

True, we have a few problems in the wee small hours, when she sleeps a little fitfully (she will soon be eight months), but we have the tools to cope and the jingle works a treat. I always know what to do in the event that she wakes up, and that is such a relief.

Putting her to bed only takes a minute or so, and she is usually off to dream land in 15 minutes. She feels very secure in her own bed.

The only thing I regret is that I didn't start the cure earlier. I also wish that I had gotten a breathing alarm earlier and started putting her to bed on her stomach. She is a stone-to-the-bone tummy sleeper. She absolutely loves it.

I think it is such a shame that children's clinics don't inform parents about breathing alarms and the advantages of tummy sleeping. It would have made life so much easier for us.

But what if the child really prefers sleeping on her back?
Three mothers from my forum describe what they did:

- *Of course you can cure a kid who sleeps on his back. Joel, three and a half months, sleeps on his back and buffing works fine. I am just careful not to lay my hand* on his chest on every fourth buff. Rocking works fine too. When I buff, I place my loosely clenched fist on the mattress, right beside his little bottom, and buff with a four beat rhythm. Joel loves that.

- I carefully raise the right leg so that knee joint makes a 90 degree angle. Then I rhythmically buff the little buttock. Fanning involves placing my spread out hand on little Annie's chest and keeping it there until she becomes sleep heavy. I don't apply any pressure but just hold my hand there lightly. She thinks it feels great and she calms down immediately.

- Jacob, who will be five soon, always slept on his back when he was little. The cure worked just fine, as did buffing. Nowadays he sleeps on his stomach more often than not. Our little girl likes sleeping on her back too. Sometimes I would try to put her to bed on her stomach, but it didn't go down that well. When she is awake, she is on her stomach as much as possible.

I just wanted to say that there is no point in obsessing over what position kids sleep in. As long as they sleep and sleep well, that's what's important.

The Goodnight Jingle

The Goodnight Jingle should be repeated four times in quick succession with only the briefest pause in between. It's rather like a cheer.

The jingle should thus consist of four verses. This can sometimes be increased to six, or even eight, if you need more time to capture the child's attention.

The jingle you eventually come up with should be rhythmic, easy to sing and provide you with the scope for every conceivable tone of voice. It should be neither too short nor too long. It should not contain the child's name, although it's tempting I know. But you are not calling the child. With the help of your jingle, *sleep* is!

The Goodnight Jingle should never be altered, although it should be modified for daytime naps so that it doesn't contain the word 'night'.

Your cure partner can choose another jingle – even another language – provided this jingle stays the same too.

My own Goodnight Jingle is a very simple one. Nightie-night-sleep-so-tight. The stress pattern is very clear: Nightie-NIGHT-sleep-so-TIGHT. During the day I say: no-more-blues-take-a-snooze. Again, the stress pattern is clear and rhythmic. No-more-BLUES-take-a-SNOOZE.

Both curers should rehearse their jingles very carefully. You can practice in the shower, outside, to music, anywhere you can listen to yourself.

And you should practice on each other. One of you fusses, whines, protests and screams, while the other jingles his or her recalcitrant better half into silence with a determination and conviction that would move mountains.

You start out strong. Verse one should be a so called 'ka-boom' jingle. Think of the carriage that you managed to grab at the last minute just before it went over the cliff! There was no time for questions or caution. In a fraction of a second, you took charge of the situation. With the same unshakable confidence, you will use the jingle to drown out your child's voice.

For the jingle to overpower the child verbally and really *calm* her, it is essential, as you understand I'm sure, that you practice loudly and conscientiously before you start the cure. Think Pavarotti!

Infants' voices have to be drowned out also for the simple reason that they become terrified by their own crying.

The jingle can be either said or sung, but in both cases the abdominal force you use should be worthy of an opera singer. It should sound decisive ('this is how things are'), happy ('everything is A OK'), joyful ('it's good to be alive'), affectionate ('you're so cute I could eat you with a spoon but that will have to wait until tomorrow'), faintly irritated ('enough is enough!') etc. There you have five variations you can practice!

When you put your child to bed on the very first evening of the *Good-Night's-Sleep Cure*, you can introduce the jingle as an ordinary, friendly good night (times four). This can be done during or just before the corrective positioning that paves the way for buffing or rocking. This will enable your child to acquaint herself with the jingle. But you will only do this once.

From then on, you jingle as you *exit*.

When you are still on the first verse, you are already on your way out, back to the bed and face to the door. When you are on verse two, you are through the door and into the hall. By verse three, you are invisible on the other side of the door (which is ajar). By the fourth and final verse, during which your voice drops and signals that the process is drawing to a close, your back is to the door as though you were heading for another part of the house.

Then it is just a question of listening. More about that in the Cheat Sheet!

As with rocking and buffing, a good rule is to make the intervals *between* jingling sessions considerably longer than the sessions themselves.

During the second night of the *Good-Night's-Sleep Cure*, you will experience a dialogue with your child. You will hear and feel how the jingle 'takes', thanks to all the hard work you have put into getting through to your child. You can adjust the tone of your voice and its strength more precisely, depending on the kind of communication that is in progress (where silence sometimes speaks louder than words).

It will become clear that the *Good-Night's-Sleep Cure* is a process. This means that it is impossible to find a way to say or sing the jingle that suits every conceivable occasion, just as it is impossible to find a way to rock or buff that suits every conceivable occasion.

Nor is it possible to make any definitive statement about how *long* you should buff, rock or jingle, or, even worse, how long a child should be 'allowed' to cry. We are talking here about *process* and *communication*. You have a euphoric experience to look forward to, since you will experience these things with your child.

The effect of the jingle is basically Pavlovian – conditioned reflex. (The bell rings and the dog starts salivating with hunger because food is served to the sound of a ringing bell.) Your child will very quickly come to associate the jingle – conditioning begins the very first night of the cure – with lie down – lie still – go to sleep – go back to sleep for the simple reason that the jingle always follows corrective positioning, rocking, buffing or fanning.

The choice of peace inducing tool(s) that precede the jingle is of course yours. Soon all that will be necessary is a jingle in passing – literally.

During the follow-up week, it is perfectly possible that all you will have to do to get your child to keel over and sleep is to jingle from your own bed.

Conditioned reflexes are not the whole story however. If it were, just a bell would do the trick.

What the jingle conveys, beyond conditioned reflexes, is a message that 'All is well' and this message can be broken down into its component parts: *peace*, followed by *security* and finally *enjoyment*.

The Confirmation Jingle

The confirmation jingle is what should follow your child to dream land.

The wording is the same as that of the goodnight jingle, but it should be soft, encouraging and, as the name implies, confirming in tone. 'You're tucked and comfy and you're going to sleep so, so well!'

The good night jingle conveys the message that it is time to sleep soundly and safely. The wolf is not at the door, and if he shows, the guns are loaded and security is guaranteed. When everything is ready, the confirmation jingle concludes the bedding procedure. Your child is drifting off or has perhaps already fallen asleep. This is the last word. The confirmation jingle slips in at the last moment and is your child's reassuring companion on her journey to the Land of Nod.

'But help! The confirmation jingle is a *disturbance!* Little Charlie was just about to fall asleep, but the confirmation got him going again!' That's how it can sound, and sometimes that's how it is.

It doesn't matter. Little Charlie needs confirmation that he is doing exactly the right thing by lying still and quiet, and feeling good about what a secure, pleasant life he has. This is a message that must be repeated whenever necessary!

In practice this means that you will have to rewind the tape a touch and go back to the powerful goodnight jingle in order to (yet again) tell little Charlie exactly what's what. Then listen, and, if necessary, provide a reminder. And listen again. And wait for the Sandman to make his entrance. And give the confirmation jingle – again. And keep going until it is accepted with contented silence.

As early as the first night of the *Good-Night's-Sleep Cure* – and certainly by the second – you will notice that your child quiets down during the good-night jingle. You can then lengthen the goodnight jingle from four to six verses (a la confirmation jingle) if you think it's appropriate, thus collapsing goodnight and confirmation into one jingle. You will no longer give the confirmation jingle separately, as it's not needed. Your child has already taken the confirmation to heart.

You are off on an exciting adventure, and the key is *listening*.

An Attitude of Supreme Confidence

At night we sleep. Everyone does. Nothing happens at night. And if you wake up, which most people do several times a night whether they remember it or not, you go back to sleep. By yourself. Because at night, nothing happens. Absolutely zip. There is nothing to do except sleep like a log.

Write this mantra on your right arm in magic marker! Or failing that, frame it and put it on the wall.

All joking aside – for I'm deadly serious – this is fundamental. This is your point of departure for an *attitude of supreme confidence*, which you should start to cultivate as soon as the starting gun for the *Good-Night's-Sleep Cure* is fired.

As you have seen, the watch word is *business-like*. There is no pleading ('Please, can't you help me out just a little?') or equivocation. There is not so much as a trace of anxiety.

The twelve-year-old on page 131, who made a habit of turning the whole household upside down with his fears and obsessions until eleven or twelve o'clock at night, found peace in only five minutes with the help of his mother's jingles (non-sequiturs every one of them). With an attitude of unshakable confidence, she managed to convey the message described above. *At night we sleep.*

Whatever worries you have out there in the world, take care of them during the day! *At night nothing happens!*

From the child's point of view, an attitude of supreme confidence translates to *security*.

This attitude of supreme confidence – of security – is the A to Z of child-care.

Insecurity is the opposite of security. Insecurity, awkward 'questioning' caution, anxiety and doubt immediately make young children nervous. To put it bluntly, they start to fear for their lives.

A firm grip on the rudder, unequivocal decisiveness, an attitude of supreme confidence – 'You are not in danger. I know how the world works. You have nothing to worry about.' – constitute nothing less than a survival guarantee to a child.

As far as a young child's sense of security goes, it's much better to be confident and wrong than diffident and right!

You are your young child's survival guarantee and you have to act like it, although at the start of the *Good-Night's-Sleep Cure* before your self-esteem is born anew, this requires a certain amount of acting talent.

- Read the chapter entitled *Peace, Security and Enjoyment* one more time. Read until you really understand what these words mean. Everything in this chapter should seem utterly self-evident by the time you are through. If it does, then I'm happy! You have laid a solid foundation for an attitude of supreme confidence.
- Read *Epilogue from Gastsjön* at the end of the book, where I talk about my personal experiences with the cure. If I managed to cure hundreds of children all by myself, you can cure one. Nothing could be simpler. Could it?
- Read through the rest of the book as well, with all the questions and answers, not least during the cure itself. There is always something more to strengthen the Attitude with. You will read with new eyes as the cure advances, no matter how many times you have read the words before.

The Attitude of Supreme Confidence is perhaps the most important strategy in the entire arsenal of the *Good-Night's-Sleep Cure*.

I am the first to understand that right now, worn down by sleep deprivation, reduced to despair, and racked by doubts about your ability to adopt any attitude at all as you are, you have difficulty grasping how in the world you could acquire the expertise and the goal-oriented decisiveness that a successful application of the *Good-Night's-Sleep Cure* requires. You are so tired that you can't think straight. Or think at all.

Don't despair! You are not alone. The perpetually perky, slept out, strong, happy, well functioning types don't seek help through the *Good-Night's-Sleep Cure*. Those who do seek help are on the verge of going under. People who aren't sick don't bother with doctors.

Remember that the *Good-Night's-Sleep Cure* is just that: a *cure*, not a method. It's there to help you, not place demands on you.

And it doesn't just cure your young child. It cures you too, along with the rest of your family.

Inexorably, consciously and actively, you must *cultivate* an attitude of supreme confidence, something that may seem as distant as outer space right now. But pay dirt is actually just around the corner. You only need to experience having a handle on everything once – that 'I-can' revelation – and the miracle happens. You will feel the self-confidence you thought was gone forever flood through you again!

And when you see how effectively the Attitude you struggled so hard to call forth works on your child – we are all lucky that young children are so easy to fool – your self-esteem will blossom, your fatigue will vanish (at least for the time being), and you will start to believe in yourself as fervently as your child does. You will find yourself in an upward spiral where the sky is the limit. You're close, believe me!

A few words from Maria M, who in 2004 became spokesperson for my then newly started parents' forum:

The way I see it, the Good-Night's-Sleep Cure *furnishes you with a mindset which enables you to actually use the tools. Without the right mindset, the tools won't work. With the right mindset, they do! With a wealth of experience behind me, I can state that that's the way things are! It is the attitude of supreme confidence that determines how you handle the tools and, ultimately, the outcome of the cure. The schedule and the tools form the foundation, but it's the mindset that actually makes things happen! The mindset is the baking powder in a recipe for sponge cake. Without the baking powder, nothing happens...*

I didn't succeed because I was so brilliant at jingling in exactly the right tone of voice in exactly the right place, or because I never deviated from the schedule by so much as a nanosecond. I succeeded because I believe in myself, in my child and in the importance of sleep for a good parent-child relationship and indeed for relationships within a family generally. We all need sleep if we are to function, think and act in a beneficial way in our everyday lives. A good sleep enables us to zero in on what is really important in life!

With the right knowledge, we all have the ability to change ourselves. Think what an asset that is! Everything we need is within us. We are not dependent on our surroundings or on experts to change our situation. I CAN DO IT MYSELF is a message that every two-year-old broadcasts to the world. We lose this belief in our own ability somewhere along the way... But if we really want to, we can find it again!

Finally, a mantra to put on your fridge right next to your MUST DO list:

If you don't call your child's night sleep into question, your child won't either.

THE CHEAT SHEET

Let's say your young child's name is Christopher and he is eight months old.

When you decide to administer the *Good-Night's-Sleep Cure*, you must commit to *seeing it through*. You can't just half-heartedly dabble and hope that the cure will take care of itself or, even worse, leave it all to your child.

Remember the joke about the grapefruit diet? 'I ate a grapefruit and then I weighed myself. I hadn't lost an ounce. What a rip-off!'

Here we sleep!

Christopher is no more to be pitied because he is to sleep all night than are his loving parents (who want nothing more in the world). There is nothing stressful or unpleasant about sleeping. To be able to sleep is – or will be – as divinely pleasurable for your child as it is – or will be – for you.

At eight months, little Chris needs approximately 14.5 hours of sleep out of every 24. Make up a schedule.

Perhaps you want him to sleep from 7.00 in the evening until 7.00 the next morning. That leaves 2.5 hours' worth of naps to be spliced into the day. Nap durations that are in sync with sleep rhythms are 5 minutes (5-minute naps can be added outside the schedule in emergencies), 20 minutes, 45 minutes, 1.5 hours, 2 hours and 3 hours.

The schedule will include four meals and Christopher will be stuffed to the gills at all of them. If necessary (at this venerable age), he will have half an hour to eat himself into a stupor (but not more) and he will get an evening top up, as much as he can get down, from Mom's breast or a bottle.

Don't worry if he doesn't eat as much as you would like. He is still too tired to eat properly. A hearty appetite will make its appearance on the third day of the *Good-Night's-Sleep Cure*, and I guarantee you that he won't have time to starve to death before then. You will be surprised when you see how little he eats after a twelve-hour stint without food!

When you draw up the schedule, make the child's existing everyday habits your guide, but write down exact times.

Stick to the schedule. You have a fifteen-minute margin of error in either direction *at the most*. Ideally, the schedule should be followed to the minute at this stage. The fifteen minute margin is dictated exclusively by your child's obvious needs.

You should start timing short daytime naps from when your child falls asleep and make sure that naps fall within the fifteen minute margin of error. If a 45-minute nap can't be squeezed in, you will have to be content with a 20-minute nap (exactly) this time.

Say good-bye to the pacifier forever. No child beyond the age of four months, at which point the urge to suck diminishes significantly, needs a pacifier. The pacifier is the original sleep destroyer and will cause even more trouble as your child gets older. Just confiscate it! *Your child will forget the pacifier in a single night.* (Provided his loving parents do of course!)

Make the clock your constant companion. It should be placed right next to the schedule you have made up, along with a pencil and paper. During the first four nights of the *Good-Night's-Sleep Cure*, write down what you do and how your child responds.

This will not only enable you to make encouraging and informative comparisons but also minimize the stress that comes with over-concentration. You know you have to get out, look at the clock and make notes.

What time did your child wake up? What did you do? How many times? What happened then? What time did he fall asleep again? When did he next wake up? What did you do this time? How did your child respond? And so on.

The bedtime laugh is the kick off. Before he goes down to sleep, little

Chris should have more fun than he has ever had in his whole life. Don't fall for all that deceptive 'wind-down-for-the-day' stuff. He should laugh until he's fit to burst!

If you are into reading stories and cuddling, detach these things from going to bed for the night. Save them for earlier in the evening or during the day when Chris is perky and alert.

If you have a choice, let the more business-like of the two of you take charge of the first two nights. Then turn the second two nights over to your better half and provide coaching and discreet tips as needed. (Just make sure the child doesn't hear you then.)

During the follow-up week, you can take turns as you both see fit.

However, you should both be present for the Good Morning Reunion, happy and raring to go!

The Message

Put your oh-so-happy child in his bed. Draw the curtains and turn off the lights. Whether you do this before or after is up to you, but the procedure should always be the same. ('Bye-bye lights. See you in the morning!')

Preferably, both Mom and Dad should be there.

Let's say that Dad is the one with the business-like edge here, so he is going to manage the first two nights. Mom says goodnight and goes on her way.

It's not a bad idea if Mom spends the night somewhere else. Dad won't be able to take care of her as well.

In the morning, you can both take part in the reunion festivities.

The third and fourth nights in our example are Mom's responsibility. Thereafter, you can alternate, even during the same night.

In a normal, friendly tone of voice, you, Dad, recite the goodnight jingle once by way of introduction, and place the child flat on his stomach without so much as a tremor. You will demonstratively place the child in a sleep inducing position: arms up, legs stretched out, and head to the right away from you. Blanket goes on, and your spread out left hand is placed over the child's back – a half fan.

With your right hand clenched in a loose fist, you immediately start to buff the little diapered bottom rhythmically and firmly, just as you have practiced with a nudge to the back for emphasis on every fourth buff.

Don't speak. The child should not hear you or see you. Keep working. Don't let up.

In the end, even though you may have quite a circus on your hands to begin with, you will feel how the little body softens up, relaxes and becomes still and hear how the child falls silent.

Before that happens, you may have to correctively position again. Do so quickly and firmly, and buff even more demonstratively. Don't get cold feet! Just do it! The penny will eventually drop (as a rule after 20 to 45 minutes).

Once Christopher is calm and quiet, and not a moment before, it will be possible for him to sleep. And this is what you must tell him, stubbornly, silently and methodically, through your actions.

As soon as your child is calm and quiet and his body has relaxed, wind down the buffing quickly and give him a final nudge with both hands spread over his whole body (the fan). The pressure should be applied for a few seconds.

Get up, turn your back and exit immediately.

On your way out begin the jingle x 4. You should be out of the room on the first verse. Go directly to verse two as you pull the door almost shut. Verse three should be said from the other side of the door (which is ajar) and on verse four (louder!) you should be on your way to wherever you're going.

Christopher may protest when you are exiting on verse one. That is allowed. Just raise your voice and speak over his! Give him all four verses at one shot or six if you feel an addition is necessary. On occasion you may have to go as high as eight. You will soon get a feel for what's needed.

Once you have fallen silent, he will react and/or pose more questions. Your task is to listen carefully.

He is 'allowed' to cry – that is the only way he can express himself, and we don't want to deny anyone the right to react. The question is *how* he cries when he reacts to the message he has received.

Perhaps neither of you has ever heard little Christopher cry before. If Mom has been in the habit of putting him to her breast as soon as he so much as peeps or has had him glued to it more or less around the clock, he has probably been pretty quiet.

The pacifier has also done its bit to ensure silence.

Now you both must learn to monitor and interpret his cries, and interpret them correctly, so that you can take the appropriate action.

Not all cries are expressions of discontent. Most cries are simply questions. 'What's going on? Is the wolf coming to get me?'

Confusion, anxiety, anger, surprise, sadness, insecurity, fear, stress, discomfort all result in different kinds of crying – just as facial expressions, not to mention word choice, chop and change in the case of an adult, depending on his or her state of mind. There is not one type of cry, any more than there is one emotional state, one human reaction or one question on everyone's mind out there in the world.

Look at the clock. What time did you leave your child's room? Write it down. Wait. *Listen.*

Are his cries gradually increasing in strength or are they gradually tapering off? The former is more likely at this early stage. But wait and listen!

Make a note of your reactions. Can you bear to permit Christopher to express himself like this? Is he really asking for help or are you the one who can't take it?

Be careful! His interests take precedence over yours! The goal is not to shut him up at any price.

The goal is to ensure that your child *finds peace.*

When you judge that it is absolutely essential to calm little Christopher down, and you feel that intervention cannot be put off any longer for his sake, then go in and repeat the message.

Without speaking, correct his position quickly and firmly: arms up with a little nudge, legs extended with a little nudge, head to the side, blanket on, spread out hand over the little back. Then start buffing again.

Don't be afraid to up the tempo and put a little more power into it. The little body should be nudged so Christopher feels it and noticeable pressure should be applied to his back with every fourth buff.

As soon as his body loosens up and he quiets down, but before he falls asleep, round off with a firm little nudge over his whole body, leave the room with verse one of the jingle, and continue with the second on the other side of the door and so on.

Pause for the reaction.

Take notes and *listen!*

Outside Christopher's room, there should be light and sound. Mozart is a good accompaniment to the *Good-Night's-Sleep Cure.*

The Reminder

Are the cries increasing in intensity? Or are they tapering off? Don't jump the gun!

If the tide seems to be rising and Christopher starts to sound truly unhappy, you will have to go in and repeat the message yet again as per the above, but in a much abbreviated form. We are talking one minute, two at the most.

The goal is still to ensure that his body relaxes and he quiets down. If he does not fall completely silent, he should at least be much calmer. Then you immediately jingle your way out.

The reminder puts the emphasis on the jingle, not the buffing.

Wait outside the door. Hold off for at least a minute or two and then start in on the next reminder jingle.

Adapt your tone of voice and the volume. Sound happy/encouraging/firm. You are looking at four rounds, or six or even eight at one shot, and make sure you keep your ears open.

Is he 'answering'? Do you sense that he is listening? Good. Wait. Practice biding your time!

The jingle x 4 (occasionally x 6 or even more occasionally x 8) takes less than 30 seconds. The time you spend *not* jingling must exceed the time you spend jingling, but you can still jingle every other minute if it's necessary.

If Christopher works himself into such a state that it's obvious that the jingle is having zero effect on him, you will have to give the message again – but keep it very short: 15–20 seconds with perhaps three rounds of buffing and an equal number of solid nudges over the little back before exiting again with the jingle (which you have now rehearsed to perfection).

Wait for the reaction again, listen again, and give the reminder jingle again – as many times as it takes.

Be ready when he finally falls silent. Then it's time for that all important conclusion.

The Confirmation

It's the same jingle, but soft, delicate and reassuring. This terminates the whole discussion. It is literally the last word.

Its tone says, 'Everything is as it should be. This is what we all do when we fall asleep. Perfect. There are no wolves as far as the eye can see. Sleep tight!'

With the first confirmation jingle, Christopher will probably start to protest, perhaps angrily, and you will probably believe that the whole enterprise has gone off the rails. He was just about to fall asleep!

But everything is as it should be. The confirmation jingle is what he will take with him when he drifts off, and he will soon calmly accept it.

However, if he recharges and starts to cry again, you will have to give him another reminder, but don't be in too much of a hurry. Listen. Let him react! There is no law against that. Quite the contrary, it is both permissible and desirable.

What is forbidden is sadness and distress.

Now that Christopher is so close to falling asleep, you are going to issue a reminder in the form of a loud, forceful jingle whose tone says that it is not a good idea to cry your way through life. 'How do you think you will be able to sleep? I don't want to hear another peep out of you! Off you go to sleep. I have got another seventeen babies out here that need help finding the peace to sleep and I have to tend to *them*. If that isn't enough, I've got eighteen cows that need milking, so I can't hang around talking to you all night. You have everything you need. Off you go to sleep!'

You have to time the confirmation perfectly, but better a touch too early than a touch too late. Your child should not have had time to fall asleep. Jingle through the door chink in a gently appreciative tone of voice. You will give a friendly confirmation x 4.

The next night, 3 or even 2 will be enough. Then you can start to merge the confirmation with the final reminder jingle.

When Christopher wakes up after his first round of sleep, you have to be quick off the mark. You cannot wait and see if he will fall back to sleep by himself. It's too early for that.

Nor must he have the chance to cry himself into a frenzy. He can cry *after* the message as a reaction or a round of new questions (see above), but he should *not* be allowed to cry when he comes to.

He has no idea what's going on when he wakes up, so he poses his first question – and this question must be answered instantly.

In light of all this, you can't count on getting any sleep yourself during the first two nights of the *Good-Night's-Sleep Cure*. Don't try sleeping on a mattress outside the door. You won't wake up in time. You have to react *instantly*.

You are in on the double and you give the message. Follow the corrective positioning routine whether it's necessary or not. Corrective positioning draws a line in the sand: all activity will now cease.

Buff quietly and efficiently, but be as brief as you possibly can. Not many rounds will be necessary – perhaps three or four. Then comes a farewell nudge and you exit with a jingle x 4.

Wait and take notes.

Issue a reminder in the form of another loud jingle but allow sufficient time for a reaction.

Wait as long as you can before you go in and buff again. If you have to buff, brief but effective is the order of the day. He must quiet down and relax. Give one last nudge and leave a little *too early*.

Remember that Christopher must have time to react to the message before he can internalize the reminder and answer it quietly and calmly.

Finish with the confirmation jingle.

Soon, perhaps as early as the next night, you will be able to merge the reminder with the confirmation, since Christopher will quiet down when you issue the reminder. You just soften your tone reassuringly and conclude the proceedings.

Continue the entire night as per the above and keep notes on the sly!

If the day is to begin at 7.00 in the morning, Christopher should be given the message/reminder/confirmation that it is still night (for him) right up to the stroke of seven.

If you have to, avail yourself of the fifteen minute margin. Within this margin, you can (preferably) wake Christopher or at least wait for contented silence. *Your child should never be taken up for the day if he is screaming.*

Time to wake up! Enter your child's bedroom with great pomp and circumstance and shout GOOD MORNING! There should be a veritable orgy of light and sound to mark the joyous reunion with much talk and merry jests.

Lift him out of bed with great fanfare! 'It's morning and ohhh, have you slept well! That's *great!*' and so on – regardless of whether Christopher has been waking up all night long yelling his head off. The fact that all your cheery ministrations seem to be pushing him towards a nervous breakdown doesn't count either. His chagrin will soon pass.

Going to bed should be fun, and it should be just as much fun to wake up to a new, exciting day!

The First Day

Follow the schedule to the letter during the day. Christopher can take his daytime naps outside on his stomach on a smooth, flat mattress. Tuck him in well with a sheet or blanket to hold him in place.

Check the clock! Wake him after exactly 20 or 45 minutes, depending on what you have planned for. (If you have decided on the longer nap option, you have the up to fifteen minute margin of error to fall back on.)

Get as much food into him as you can, but feedings should not last longer than half an hour. Prune puree, a laxative, is recommended for dessert every day during the *Good-Night's-Sleep Cure*. Shoot for one jar a day.

Keep him awake by any means necessary during those periods when he is supposed to be awake!

Little Chris is going to be very tired today.

The Second Night

The bedding procedure will go a lot faster. Keep notes and compare with the previous night.

Take care not to buff a second longer than is absolutely necessary so that you don't get stuck in the 'buffing trap'. For Christopher is actually starting to like being buffed and would be only too pleased if you kept up the good work! Why not all night?

Rescue him from this delusion! He will only be buffed to convey the all important *message* that accompanies a happy bedtime. The jingle will do the rest.

But don't allow yourself to fixate on the jingle either. Don't over-focus on the child. Once you have banished the wolves of anxiety, *move away from the door*.

From the second night on, buffing should be restricted to crisis situations. And I mean Crisis with a capital C. Buff as briefly, efficiently and infrequently as you possibly can.

Ideally, the jingle should take over completely during this second night.

After the first night, it is not necessary to buff or jingle until the child is completely silent. There is nothing dangerous or negative about being angry, which, for now, is probably what Christopher will be at regular (and irregular) intervals.

After the first night, you will start jingling without entering the child's room when he wakes up after having slept for a while. But bide your time and listen! When, in spite of everything, you are about to rush in and buff, *that's* the time to jingle.

Little Christopher will also manage to fall asleep again by himself the odd time without your having to do anything at all. You won't even have time to jingle before peace descends. And won't that be fabulous!

The focus this night is thus the jingle, the reminder jingle, which reminds the child of the message that has been conveyed. 'The sun has gone down, and now you are going to sleep soundly. The wolf won't get you because I am standing guard. Nothing bad is going to happen to you so you can relax,' is what you are expressing in the tone and volume of your voice.

You will of course adapt your tone, just as you did on the first night, to the child's way of posing questions so that the answer hits home.

Don't forget the confirmation jingle! During this second night, your goal is that the confirmation jingle not be followed by protests. Repeat the jingle as needed so that it really is the last word.

Since all contact will now cease, you may start to worry about how he is actually lying. Is he on top of the covers? Is he cold?

When he has been asleep for ten minutes – not 20 – you can quickly sneak in and throw an extra blanket over him. He is probably lying diagonally across the foot of the bed curled up in a ball. Leave him be! Don't take any risks at this stage of the game.

The next night you will be able to reposition him quickly in his bed if necessary (after ten minutes, not twenty) without his noticing.

The Second Day

Don't take any liberties with the schedule at this stage, no matter how tough you think it is to stick to it. Always be prepared. Always stay one step ahead. The schedule is Holy Writ.

The entire enterprise stands or falls by the timetable you have decided on.

This is as true for the days as it is for the nights. Everything is dependent on everything else.

The child's appetite should start to improve today (although perhaps not in the morning). Overtiredness begins to give way to healthy sleepiness. Little Chris will probably be rubbing his eyes and yawning his way through the day, which is a good sign!

The Third Night

Same procedure as the second night, but buffing goes!

During the bedding procedure itself, you, Mom, assuming as we are that you are taking over, can buff delicately just for emphasis, but you can also content yourself with fanning (after a demonstrative round of corrective positioning) and holding the child in place for a few seconds.

Then exit with a jingle and don't hang around on the threshold.

At this point, the reminder jingle starts to work on its own. It is followed by – and ultimately merged with – the confirmation jingle. The reactions, protests and/or questions will be of significantly shorter duration or will disappear entirely. The child asks, is answered and is content with that.

Little Christopher doesn't sound particularly unhappy now. Actually, he doesn't sound unhappy at all. Just the opposite in fact! The little angel spews 'oaths' you had no idea he knew!

But angry 'oaths' and profane 'words' are better than emotional break-downs. Christopher is starting to perceive the message. He may, for example, get mightily ticked off because he *wants* to sleep but *can't*, at least not right away. That he finds really irritating!

You can now sleep a little yourself between rounds (in an adjacent room so that you will hear immediately if and when he wakes up). You can then race for the door and listen, ready to jingle if required.

This night, it is possible that Christopher will fall back to sleep sev-eral times all by himself. Consequently, it is permitted to hold back a little while before you jingle – provided he isn't crying.

Note my use of the word *crying!* Whines and grumbles don't count. Tonight is the night he puts crying behind him!

The Third Day

By now little Chris has logged more hours in total and for longer continuous periods than ever before. He has often not even really come to, but has drifted back to sleep by himself.

You're on the right track! Good work!

Today he is much perkier. He whines less but is still sleepy. He is eating more than he ever has in his life (and this can lead to constipation, so keep giving him the prune purée). The dark circles under his eyes are beginning to disappear. His pallid face takes on a little color.

Respect the schedule scrupulously! The *Good-Night's-Sleep Cure*'s four 24-hour periods and the follow-up week's seven is not the time for changes and certainly not schedule changes.

Peace, simplicity and cast iron predictability are what must be cultivated now.

If these three nights and days have all been managed as they should, today is the day you will witness a metamorphosis. The child will literally bloom. His cheeks are rosy, his eyes crystal clear, and a smile and a laugh are never far away. Christopher is finally getting his strength – I left the word 'back' out on purpose because he has never had the strength that was his due. He has been running on empty his whole life.

But now you can both claim you reward, just as Christopher can. With sound sleep and tranquil routines, the child blossoms like a flower in the sun right before your eyes. It is truly a sight to behold!

By the fourth day and night the schedule really begins to take root. Suddenly the days and nights can be planned and foreseen. This confers enormous advantages, as you will see. You know what is going to happen and when, and so does your child. You have assumed your roles as leaders. You know what you are doing and why, and little Christopher constantly receives reassuring confirmation of that fact. His relief over your confidence is impossible to miss.

And your child will be a tremendous help to you, once his relief enters the picture. And this relief manifests itself when the routines are written in stone and may not be questioned.

You may find yourself wondering why he is suddenly whining. You then cast a glance at the clock and the schedule and exclaim, 'His midday nap is in five minutes. That's why!'

Never again will you fall into that slough of puzzled insecurity. Life becomes simple and perpetually agreeable. No more crying, no more whining.

It may well happen that one point or other in the program will run into difficulties for a couple of weeks. Usually it involves one of the daytime naps.

Just follow the schedule unwaveringly and this too shall pass.

The most important thing is not that little Christopher sleeps every minute he is 'supposed to'. The most important thing is that he is supplied with the prerequisites to do so!

During the night, you may still have to issue the odd reminder – the wee small hours, the so called hour of the wolf, between 4.00 and 6.00 a.m. can be problematic for a while yet.

Stay calm. If you rush in, buff and generally carry on, you are saying through your actions 1) the wolf is at the door or, 2) morning has come – neither of which is true. So, *no through traffic!*

Give Christopher a cheerful, matter-of-fact, explanatory jingle if and when he wakes up during 'the hour of the wolf' and do it quick – i.e. before he starts to scream. Then be quiet. You can make other sounds around the house or you can just go back to bed.

Mozart and Strauss are always trusty companions. (N.B. Only instrumental pieces. Nothing with lyrics.)

Now we are looking at a bedding procedure that takes two minutes at the most, daytime naps included.

You can invite people home and when the time comes, simply tell your guests, 'I'm just going to put Christopher to bed.' They will all think that you'll be out of circulation for a couple of hours, but you're back before they've had time to so much as stretch their legs. 'Where were we?' you say. Whereupon everybody thunders, 'He's asleep *already?* But he didn't even look tired!'

The reminders will become short one-time events, and you must bear in mind that *in order for Christopher to continue to move forward, you have got to step back – first,* and continuously so.

So, be on guard against a tendency to over-focus on your child! Train yourselves to leave him in peace. He *wants* to sleep. He doesn't want you hanging over him, and he will let you know in no uncertain terms if you persist in doing so.

The Follow-up Week

The follow-up week after the *Good-Night's-Sleep Cure*'s first four days and nights ensures that all these novelties become routine.

Now that the vicious cycle has been broken, a benevolent one replaces it. You have succeeded in giving your child peace. You have helped Christopher find his way to a peaceful place time after time after time. Now he dares to fall asleep and go back to sleep all by himself.

You have done a sterling job! Congratulations!

But you're not done yet.

If you have skipped forward to The Cheat Sheet because it seemed to be the shortest route, you would be well advised to carefully study the chapter on *Security*. Otherwise, you run the risk of running aground just when you thought the home port was in sight.

The follow-up week should be nothing if not tranquil. The days and nights should be as identical as possible. This is not the right time for trips, impression filled visits, novel, disorienting activities or nights away from home.

The world has to be little before it can be large, and this is especially true during the *Good-Night's-Sleep Cure*.

Little Christopher has been made privy to a fair amount of revolutionary information. Now he has to internalize it.

And then he will understand that every day is going to be as glorious as the last, something that he doesn't dare hope for some evenings (which may cause him to fall apart).

So let nothing stand in the way of the bedtime laugh and the joyous, fun filled morning reunions! When time and experience have left their marks, and Christopher has truly understood that the fun doesn't end at bedtime but comes back every morning, he will think it's super to be put to bed and to go to sleep.

During the follow-up week, if not before, young children usually begin to sleep the whole night through.

It is equally common for illness to strike the little angels at this point. Latent ailments manifest themselves when the child has the strength to cope with them. These ailments flare up – and then disappear.

Don't let them influence your attitude of supreme confidence!

This attitude says that being sick is no fun, but *nothing is wrong and no danger threatens.*

Anything that may happen can be dealt with in bed if you have a sick, feverish child to deal with. This includes changing diapers, giving water and comfort (but not anxiety) and even changing sheets.

It sounds brutal, but the rule is this: Don't pick the child up unless you have to take her to the ER!

With all this newfound strength, Christopher's immune system will soon crank into high gear.

You will enter a zombie-like state when you realize that you can actually count on being able to sleep at night. People will ask you, 'Why are you so tired? You can sleep now!' 'Exactly!' you will reply.

Good Luck!

Remember that anxiety is always the villain in the piece when it comes to childcare. Do not constantly impose your anxious presence on your child in the mistaken belief that he cannot live without it!

Anxiety raises fear in the child's mind, and no little kid can stand that. (Neither can big ones for that matter.) Without exception, the result will be protests.

You can never expect guidance from an infant. The child is waiting frantically for guidance from you.

Don't make the mistake of standing glued to your child's bedside and constantly buffing when it is no longer necessary. The child has gotten the message, something that usually happens during the first night or, at the latest, the second. Jingle loudly and calmly without going in.

In emergencies you can quickly and silently reposition the child, hold him in place for a few seconds with both hands (fanning) and then immediately exit with a jingle. As soon as you relieve the pressure, your eyes are on the door, not the child.

Don't hang around! All you are doing is *disturbing him.*

Best of luck with your newly acquired, truly reassuring, firm hand! Which little Christopher will come to appreciate, since he will be able to devote his new found energy to growing, developing and being happy – secure in the knowledge that from now on he doesn't have to look out for his own interests in this world. That is a task that he is just not up to.

With simple determination, with the goal of a good sleep for everyone constantly in mind, and with patience and confidence in your child and yourselves, you will easily do what has to be done to achieve rapid and lasting results.

Rome wasn't built in a day and you must resign yourselves to the fact that your work in progress will take about four weeks before every point in the program will be sitting solidly. Rome rose to greatness and withstood the proverbial slings and arrows of outrageous fortune. It is not called the eternal city for nothing!

With the *Good-Night's-Sleep Cure*, you will give Christopher a wholesome, sound, secure sleep, the kind of sleep he *really wants.* It's the kind of sleep that is not placed in jeopardy by colds or teething. It will give him true security, which will soon become a part of him.

With the *Good-Night's-Sleep Cure*, you are giving your child a liberating, predictable existence, an existence free from sleep deprivation and poor appetite, as well as prodigious freedom of movement for all of you (provided that you stick to the timetable).

Good sleep means a good life, a life where *joie de vivre* gets the space it deserves. It is the most precious gift you can give your child.

And it's not a bad present to give yourselves either!

HOW LITTLE LARRY, THREE AND A HALF MONTHS, FOUND HIS WAY TO A GOOD NIGHT'S SLEEP: AN EMAIL EXCHANGE

MOM AND DAD

Since insecurity gets its claws into everyone from time to time (not good!), we wanted to check with you to make sure we were on the right track so that we don't end up just 'trying out' new sleep habits but really make them stick.

Larry, three and a half months, is going to be moved to a crib and will start to sleep through the night. We thought it was best to contact you directly (so that we don't start asking Larry questions). The breathing alarm arrived by mail today.

Here is Larry's schedule:

6.00 a.m. Food (x 2), morning wash, morning housework (with Dad)

7.00 a.m. Top up and nap

9.00 a.m. Food (x 2), diaper change, solitary games, morning activities (with Mom)

11.00 a.m. Top up, nap outdoors

1.00 p.m. Food (x 2), diaper, activities (participates in doing dishes, preparing meals, reading)

3.00 p.m. Top up, nap outdoors

5.00 p.m. Food (x 2) diaper change, activities

7.00 p.m. Awake, socializing

8.00 p.m. Food (x 2) and evening bath

9.00–9.30 p.m. Top up and bedtime

We have been following this schedule for about a month. Larry is always awake for around 9 hours out of every 24. I always offer two rounds of food + a top up. Larry has virtually stopped taking food during round two. Should I try to dispense with the top up?

The meal at 8.00 p.m. has begun to run into problems too. He is not interested in food. He just turns his head away and sometimes starts to cry. Our big little lad (7.5 kg) is still on breast milk only.

On to sleep. So far, we have 'rocked' him to sleep. And we have continued to rock when he has woken up at night. On those occasions when he has cried/asked questions, we've picked him up (hmm, I guess the wolf got in!).

The last few nights, it has taken about half an hour to rock him to sleep, and then we have rocked him several times (more than several actually) during the wee small hours, that 'hour of the wolf'.

Here is what we are planning:
We have borrowed a crib. Larry has never slept in one before. Do you think it's a good idea to bring a crib into the picture the same night that we stop rocking him and introduce stomach sleeping (which he is already trying accomplish on his own)? Or are we introducing too much too soon? Our carriage seems too cramped for stomach sleeping.

The evening bath and fun & games with both Mom and Dad start at 8.00.

We feed him just before 9.00. As for the other meals, he usually goes to sleep right after the top up, but he rarely does so after the 9.00 p.m. meal. Sometimes I think he is too alert and sometimes I think he is too tired.

We position him correctively, place both hands on his back, apply a little light pressure and leave with a goodnight jingle – one at the bedside, one on the way out, and one more at the chink in the door.

Now we get to the things we're not sure about. When and how should we intervene?
1. If he starts to bang his head against the mattress and ask a lot of questions, we wait a little while and then jingle through the chink in the door when Larry is quiet but not yet asleep.

2. *If he starts to cry himself into a panic, we jingle first, position correctively and buff as long as it takes until he is quiet but not yet asleep. Then we jingle again. If he wakes up, we start all over.*
3. *If he wants answers to questions in the middle of the night, I jingle as soon as he wakes up. If that doesn't help, we buff again and round off with a jingle.*
4. *If he wakes up during the second or third night, hopefully a jingle will be sufficient. If he starts to cry himself into a panic, we position correctively and buff (in emergencies).*

Perhaps we sound a little unsure of ourselves, but we are convinced that we will succeed in showing our son how he can find peace and sleep soundly.

ANNA

It sounds as though you are superbly motivated and determined, and I am certain that everything will go just swimmingly! As long as you bear in mind that the *Good-Night's-Sleep Cure* is a process – five steps forward and two back sometimes – you will keep the wolf at bay. You will know what you are doing and you won't worry.

Yes, you should dispense with the top up now. He is big enough to eat his fill at one sitting.

He should also begin to fall asleep by himself. He should no longer need a knock-me-out top up. So see to it that he gets down as much as possible during the two rounds (or three or four if you like), but it should take no more than an hour! As things stand now, according to the schedule you showed me, he is actually eating every 90 minutes throughout the day, which means ten meals a day! He no longer needs that.

Spread out the meals, and that, in combination with a good night's sleep, will enable Larry to eat with a much better appetite at every meal. That in turn, although it seems paradoxical, will ensure that Larry won't continue to gain weight so rapidly.

In the evening however, he can (and should) be given a final top up before bed, before or after the bedtime laugh, whichever you prefer. The interval between the last meal and the top up won't be more than an hour.

Larry stays up a little too late. (Great social participation in this schedule!) If he is up for the day at six, he should go to bed at eight in the evening if you are shooting for a ten-hour night. (In only a couple of weeks, he will be mature enough for a twelve-hour night.) So think about that before you finalize the schedule! The last meal runs into problems now because he is just too tired that late in the evening. He sometimes gets his second wind and gets 'perky', or he gets overtired. This is not the objective. Larry doesn't have the strength for it in the long run.

Think about a schedule like the following (just a suggestion):

6.00 a.m. to 7.00 a.m. Feeding
8.30 a.m. to 10.00 a.m. Nap 1.5 hours
10.00 a.m. to 11.00 a.m. Feeding
12.00 noon to 2.00 p.m. Midday nap 2 hours
2.00 p.m. to 3.00 p.m. Feeding
4.00 p.m. to 5.30 p.m. Nap 1.5 hours
5.30 p.m. to 6.30 p.m. Feeding
7.00 p.m. Bath
7.30 p.m. Evening top up and bedtime laugh
8.00 p.m. Down for the night

As you see, he is eating right after every nap and learns to fall asleep by himself during these naps, right after social participation. Eating is not the last thing he does.

This suggested schedule also allows for 15 hours of sleep out of 24, just as yours does. It's possible that he will take an extra quarter of an hour every now and then if he gets the chance. You can always cut him fifteen minutes of slack (or five or ten, but not more than fifteen) if he doesn't want to wake up right on time.

The fifteen minute margin – in both directions – enables you to be sensitive to your child's wishes without compromising the fixed routines.

Introduce all the changes at once! The clearer you are from the start, the easier it is for Larry to learn the new drill.

He will be confused at first, but on the second night, he will start to believe that that's the way 'things have always been'. (You are not still using a pacifier I trust. If you are, it can go at the same time! Larry will forget all about it in one night.)

You will begin by buffing. It is unavoidable if you have been rocking up to now. The little body must be allowed to benefit from those 'nudges'. Practice your technique on each other!

First comes demonstrative corrective positioning. Then start to buff in silence. This will take anywhere from 20 to 45 minutes the first time you do it, but it will never take that long again! When he relaxes and falls silent, exit promptly with a jingle.

Preferably, whoever takes the first two nights (i.e. the most business-like of the two of you) should be out the door on the first 'verse', *never* at the bedside. The rest of the jingle should be said outside the door (not through the chink), which is ajar but only open a tiny crack.

1. It is very important to jingle immediately in answer to his questions the minute he wakes up and asks them. Don't let him even get close to crying himself into a panic. It is just as important to listen patiently and not be in too much of a hurry to start the next jingle. The rule on the first night is this: the time you spend *not* jingling must exceed the time you spend jingling. Let me explain. If you immediately jingle x 4 or x 6 or even occasionally x 8 at one shot, expecting the jingle to 'hit home' (which it won't the first time), this will take perhaps 30 seconds. You will *not* jingle for at least a minute. This is your game plan during the first night when the confusion is total! Then you will jingle less and less frequently, and the intervals between rounds will become longer and longer.

2. If he screams himself into a frenzy in spite of the jingles and needs help to calm down, reposition quickly, silently and firmly, and buff again until he is relaxed and quiet. Then leave immediately. Don't linger by

the bedside. You can round off with a little pressure over his back. Then get up and head for the door, jingling as you exit. Splice in the confirmation jingle at exactly the right moment so that Larry takes it with him into dream land. If he protests (which he will on and off the first night), start over with the reminder – but take your time. Don't jump the gun! Wait for the right moment before you start the confirmation. Continue until the confirmation jingle has the last word.

3. Yes, plus a confirmation.
4. Yes, the jingle gradually takes over completely, and he should also be given the chance to fall back to sleep by himself after grumbles, whimpers etc., so you no longer have to be as quick off the mark with the jingle. Buffing disappears, and in emergencies you have corrective positioning to fall back on, followed by a brief fanning session and a jingle on the way out. You can then buff if you feel you have to draw the line when you put Larry down for the night – just a few rounds to make sure he gets the message if you think it is appropriate, instead of being content with corrective positioning. But we are talking no more than three or four seconds!

Whatever you do, you must conclude as quickly as you possibly can (better too early than too late). It's a question of constantly thinking things out. It's a good idea to have a pencil, paper and a clock in the kitchen, where you can keep notes on what happened at what time, so you can't hang around in Larry's room!

As soon as he relaxes and quiets down – complete silence should reign the first night, but this is not necessary on the second – you are out of there. If you think in terms of operating outside the child's room instead of inside, soon your child will catch on and will not cry to get you *into* the room but to keep the wolf *out*. Thus, you can go back to keeping the wolf at bay from outside the child's room rather than trying to do so from inside, which of course is disturbing.

Remember that the *Good-Night's-Sleep Cure* is a process – that's why it's both fun and useful to keep a record of the course of events. Thus, the drill won't be exactly the same night after night (as we saw above with the jingling for example) and we can't predict exactly how long a child should be 'allowed' to cry before it is appropriate to intervene with a jingle. (As far as I'm concerned, no child should cry at all, apart from the very first time I buff on the first night. I am the one who should be able to stop the crying by conveying sufficiently reassuring messages. The child shouldn't have to do it for me.)

There are new challenges every night. The child poses questions differently and these questions require different answers or sometimes no answers at all. Sometimes the child answers these questions himself... It's a wonderfully exciting adventure! You will become tremendously adept at listening and knowing exactly what you should do – and what you shouldn't do!

Don't make the mistake of obsessing over how things 'should' be because there are so many variables. Take one step at a time. First, Larry has to learn to perceive the message. The penny has to drop, the penny that says, 'It is not dangerous to fall asleep on your own!'

Once he has understood that, then the dialogue changes. It will feel so delightful! You will have a steady hand on the tiller, and you will be able to pull back and have more and more faith in him as you see and feel that he both can and really *wants* to sleep well.

But the first night and often the second as well *are* difficult and involve much running back and forth, since the little angel has not yet understood quite what all this is in aid of. This is inevitable. That's why I try to prepare people for two truly sleepless nights. Whoever is in charge should not count on being able to go to bed at all, but must be ready and able to answer the child's questions *immediately* all night long. On the third night, it is usually possible to sleep on and off, often for many hours at a stretch.

To conclude: *The Good-Night's-Sleep Cure* encompasses not only four days and nights, but also a tranquil and methodical follow-up week. It is during this follow-up week that most little angels start to sleep continuously through the night. However, during the first four days and nights, they do start to fall back to sleep by themselves if and when they wake up – and that's what we were aiming for, wasn't it? No one is afraid of the big, bad wolf anymore!

So be patient and believe in your child! Pull back more and more, and never disturb your child unless it is absolutely necessary. Remember that the all important message is this: *At night nothing happens.*

At the beginning, you can make the crib less spacious with a couple of tightly rolled baby blankets to hem him in a little, but nothing too soft and nothing too high up. He must be able to move his head from side to side.

MOM AND DAD
We have completed the cure and the follow-up week. It went pretty well for the most part. Here are some of our notes:

Night 1
8.15 p.m.
The future late sleeper was repositioned and immediately began to ask questions. (These questions increased both in frequency and volume.) I buffed for 25 minutes until he was completely relaxed physically but still awake. (All the while I was thinking, 'This will go faster the next time, this will go faster the next time...') I made a quick exit, jingling as I left. He was soon in full swing again, but I held off a little while, and he gradually simmered down! Then it was time for the confirmation jingle and then he went to sleep!

11.35 p.m.
Woke up. I jingled immediately. Listened. The protests came thick and fast, so I went in and buffed. Jingled again. Buffed again. Jingled again. (Took about 10 minutes.)
1.50 a.m.
Jingled. Buffed. Jingled. Buffed. Jingled. Buffed. Jingled = too many times. I think I intervened too quickly. (I was afraid he was about to wake the neighbors.)

4.00 a.m. to 6.00 a.m.
He woke up several times, laughed in his sleep, sucked his thumb... I jingled once (5.00) and was answered with silence.

6.00 a.m.
Super(lative) morning.
We tried to live according to the 'load the gun in the hall' theory i.e. out as fast as possible.

Nights 2 and 3 *went well. Larry woke up a couple of times but he usually fell back to sleep himself.*

Nights 4–6 *went brilliantly. He pretty well slept right through. When he woke up, he talked to himself a little, wiggled around in his bed and then heaved a deep sigh that seemed to say, 'Might as well go back to sleep. Nothing happening around here anyway!'*

Right now, it seems as though his night sleep is veering off course again. He wakes up several times a night. Last night I jingled. I haven't had to do that for quite a while. Sometimes he even sobs. I don't know what we have done wrong!

Naps during the day still aren't going well. He seldom sleeps more than 45 minutes when he should be sleeping 1.5 hours. The nap between 4.00 p.m. and 5.30 p.m. is especially tough. Outdoor naps work better, but indoors it is difficult to get him to go to sleep (and to go back to sleep) during the day. Maybe the day-time naps will get easier in a couple of weeks when the schedule has really had a chance to sink in.

The penny hasn't really dropped yet, but we are hoping that with a little time and patience it eventually will.

When our friends talk about the Cry-It-Out Method, it gives us a good feeling to know that we didn't fall into the trap of using that simplistic and horrible escape hatch. Instead we have used your method, which demands energy, trust, love, time and commitment. We feel as though we have given our son something that will benefit him all his life.

Let's take a look at the schedule:
6.00 a.m. to 7.00 a.m. Feeding, feeding and more feeding
8.00 a.m. to 9.30 a.m. Nap 1.5 hours
9.30 a.m. to 10.30 a.m. Feeding
12.00 noon to 2.00 p.m. Nap 2 hours
2.00 p.m. to 3.00 p.m. Feeding
4.00 p.m. to 5.30 p.m. Nap 1.5 hours
5.30 p.m. to 6.30 p.m. Feeding

7.00 p.m. Bath
7.30 p.m. Bedtime top up
8.00 p.m. Bedtime laugh and down for the night

ANNA

You have done a superb job! And so has little Larry. He is one smart kid! Not all little angels get the message as fast as he has. Things have gone brilliantly and I am very proud of all three of you.

Now it is just a question of staying the course without looking back or even sideways. Just keep your mind facing front. The fact that he has been a little more wakeful and even had the odd bout of crying is of course no fun for anybody, but it is nothing unusual and will soon pass.

For one thing, he is sleeping so much more than he used to that he thinks he is slept out, which he isn't. (This has perhaps been most noticeable during the day up to now. It will soon pass too.)

For another, the occasional relapse goes with the territory. A child can get all this out of his system in one truly terrible night, or, in exceptional cases, draw the process out over several. It seems as though young children have to immerse themselves one last time in that confusion and insecurity that once was their lot in life in order to come to the conclusion that peace reigns; the wolf isn't coming for them.

The *Good-Night's-Sleep Cure* requires a certain amount of time, and not until the follow-up week is done can we count on a certain degree of stability. With time, experiences pile up in the child's mind.

Simply put, little Larry must figure some things out by himself. 'Nothing's happening! I really can sleep! And nothing's happening now either!' It takes time for all of us to acquire reliable experience and take it to heart.

So whatever you do, don't think that just because 'something is going on', something must be wrong. The cure is a process – and that can mean five steps forward and two steps back. So stay the course, and if you have to, read up again so that you know exactly what you are doing and why, and don't allow yourself to feel even a whisper of anxiety. (Your anxiety = the wolf.)

So you have adopted the schedule I suggested? (I'm blushing with pride!) If you introduced everything at once a little less than two weeks ago, it should have sunk in relatively well I think, but the daytime naps are still a problem.

The 45-minute nap is a classic and is ideally suited to a natural sleep rhythm.

When he wakes up, let him be for as long as you can and jingle as little as possible. Limit yourself to one confirmation jingle when he decides to go back to sleep and one generous reminder if and when he takes it into his head *not* to go back to sleep. What's important now is not whether he sleeps every single minute that he is supposed to, but that he has the prerequisites to do so. So give him these prerequisites and make sure they stick!

And be consistent with locations until everything solidifies. If you have decided he is to take a certain nap in the carriage, it should be the same nap every day. Follow the same procedure with the bed indoors. Watch the clock and don't exceed the fifteen minute margin (ideally stay well within it). Soldier on faithfully and methodically, and disturb him as little as possible.

You will manage brilliantly and the road ahead is straight and clear! If you do hit a bump, stay cool. There is a possibility that that last nap will have to be cut to 45 minutes. If, for a whole week (no less), he stubbornly demonstrates that he has real problems managing the entire 1.5 hours and you can't persuade him otherwise, then revise the schedule as necessary.

Thank you for your warm and thought provoking words at the end! Yes, the *Good-Night's-Sleep Cure* is more than a method or a mere technique. It is a philosophy of life. Successfully administered, it constitutes a point of departure with regard to both children and parenthood that is diametrically opposed to that which is so distressingly current in the Western world today.

MOM AND DAD

The penny really is starting to drop! Life with a baby is now absolutely fantastic.

During the last week, Larry's night sleep has improved and stabilized. The last three nights, he has barely surfaced at all. Sometimes he wiggles around a little in his bed, but he goes back to sleep pretty quickly. Last night he had a nasty dream (poor lad) and cried a little.

The wee small hours (4.00–6.00 a.m.) were a bit of a problem for about two and a half weeks. But now, as we said, we've made quite a bit of progress. If someone had told me a month ago that when Larry turned four months, he would be sleeping 10 hours a night and going to sleep by himself to boot, I would never have believed it.

Patience and confidence in your child are two important ingredients in the Good-Night's-Sleep Cure in our opinion.

Larry is happy and looks forward to everything because everything is so much fun. One of our acquaintances exclaimed delightedly, 'He's one happy little camper!'

That reminds me, there is something I have to tell you... You once wrote that little people can't be too careful when choosing their parents. Some people are dumb, some people are dumber and some people are brain dead. The other night, I think I qualified for the third category.

I was woken up by Larry wiggling around in his bed, so I assumed it was morning. I looked at the clock and it was 5.45. I stretched, turned on the light and launched into my happy-happy-joy-joy morning routine. Larry woke up. Suddenly, I got the feeling that something was wrong. Both Larry and my husband looked so sleepy. Then my husband said, 'What are you doing? It's only 3.00 a.m.!' Was he right or was he right...

The daytime naps have also started to go better. Little Larry has actually slept for 1.5 hours between 4.00 and 5.30 p.m. several times now. He frequently wakes up after 45 minutes, but he usually falls back to sleep. The schedule is working well I think. He seems to have gotten used to the timetable. We feel like traitors if we have to deviate from it!

To conclude:
When Larry was just over four months, it was time to introduce the twelve-hour night. It happened to coincide with moving the clocks forward, so we piggybacked on daylight saving and the little man got his twelve-hour night when the rest of the country had to get up an hour earlier. We changed the schedule so that the night ran from 7.30 to 7.30, and that's how it's been ever since.

Suddenly we had a son who slept all night and was in a good mood all day.

If we compare our lives before and after the cure, it really is chalk and cheese. My husband and I had masses of adult time together and we felt so much more secure in our roles as parents.

All three of us got our lives back. Larry had a profound sense of security that we were proud to have given him. We also noticed physical improvements. He was so much more alert and healthy. (He was three years old before he got his first real bout of flu complete with fever.)

No one ever questioned his daytime routines again. That freed up – and continues to free up – so much energy for other things. He has time to prepare food, make beds, vacuum, wash cars and so much else. We have quite an actively partaking assistant in our household!

With that I'd like to say that the Good-Night's-Sleep Cure *is about so much more than just sleep. Life should be well lived!*

To this day, I still silently thank the wisdom contained in Anna's Good-Night's-Sleep Cure. *Were it not for that, our son would certainly have grown up plagued by sleep deprivation and complaining parents. Today he loves to snuggle down in his bed, adjust his pillow carefully, and then drop off to sleep.*

To be able to see and enjoy a child who has had his basic needs fulfilled and who can devote himself to exploring the world gives you a taste for more. When Larry was barely one and a half years old, he got a little brother!

Postscript

Today Larry turns four! It's been a little over three and a half years since we cured him. In all this time, he has only woken up three times that we have noticed.

The first time, he was around six months (May 2004) and was struggling with his first cold. I remember he was unhappy and had a very stuffy nose.

The second time was in connection with the eight-month anxiety (July 2004). He screamed his head off for an hour after being put to bed and then fell asleep.

The third time was at the beginning of his terrible two's (November 2006). He cried in the middle of the night and babbled about horses with pink manes jumping up on his bed.

On all three occasions, I first repositioned him (to check that nothing external was wrong) and then jingled. I would go in only once and then rely on the jingle.

The boys have the jingle in the bones. We still use it at bed time. If I am sometimes distracted and forget, they immediately pipe up, 'Mom, you forgot to say night-night...'

So it cannot be denied that this particular tool continues to function long after the cure!

Sometimes I ask myself how our nights would have been if we hadn't cured Larry... I don't even want to think about it.

The Good-Night's-Sleep Cure has been much more than merely useful. It was our point of departure when we were at one of life's crossroads. As a result, we decided to let the world stay small for little people until they get big.

'Big' things are happening to them anyway. Larry, for example, has just graduated from a crib to a junior size bed. I can state that, thus far, he has never climbed out of bed at night (neither has his little brother for that matter).

Last autumn, it was time for young master Larry to broaden his horizons. He now takes part in a children's club two afternoons a week. There are eight kids aged between three and a half and four and a half. They get together and busy themselves with playing and eating snacks, and are supervised by two group leaders. I think it is a superb arrangement because:

- The kids must be at least three to join
- The sessions are just the right length
- Everyone in the group was (is) a first-time participant
- There is more than enough staff
- The fee for a term is €35

And any day now, a little brother or a little sister will be arriving!

Pia, licensed Good-Night's-Sleep Curer, Finland.

THE GOOD-NIGHT'S-SLEEP CURE:
QUESTIONS AND ANSWERS

No support
My husband thinks that we should pick Jacob up whenever he cries, and I buff and jingle, buff and jingle. I feel so hopeless because I get no support at all from my husband.

As one mother said to her husband, 'Fine, pick him up, but you take the night shifts from now on!' – which of course wasn't what he had in mind.

During the first two nights of the *Good-Night's-Sleep Cure*, it is really beneficial to be able to concentrate on the task of calming the child and breaking old sleep deprivation patterns without having to contend with complaints and skepticism from your surroundings. Consequently, you should see to it that you are alone with the child so that you can get on with the job in peace without having to explain to the world that you know what you're doing. The people around you will see the results soon enough, and they usually have enough sense to appreciate them – *then*.

The hour of the wolf
Anne, five months, wakes up every morning between 4.00 and 4.30. Can I give her formula when I change her diaper? She falls back to sleep beautifully, sleeps until 7.00, and then I do the good-morning routine.

Unfortunately, she will not suddenly start sleeping through that meal of her own accord and go on sleeping until seven. Rather, the day will come when she won't go back to sleep after being fed. At that point, you can either start the day at four or implement the *Good-Night's-Sleep Cure* fully.

Waking up during the hour of the wolf (between four and six in the morning) can continue for a long time – sometimes several weeks. The child wakes up and thinks she is slept out (which she isn't). She proceeds to play and babble and maybe even sing, and then she falls apart because morning 'never' comes. If you provide entertainment in the form of a bottle, a diaper change, or your mere presence, at least *something* is happening, which means the day has begun! This in turn usually leads to the nights becoming shorter and shorter. If you pick up a child in the midst of the cure even half an hour too early, then as surely as day follows night, the next morning will start half an hour early too, and before you know it, you are right back to where you started from.

It is all a question of focusing on and conveying the over-arching message: *At night nothing happens.*

The important thing is that the child goes back to sleep during the hour of the wolf, if only for five minutes. Even a nap that brief will enable the child to bridge the gap and cut down the waking time until she finally sleeps through the hour of the wolf completely.

It's a delicate balancing act. On the one hand, you've got to convince the child that it is appropriate to sleep a little longer. The child is, after all, asking a question, and questions have to be answered. On the other, you should not disturb the child and start entertaining her. *At night everyone sleeps. At night nothing happens.*

You can nip this problem in the bud. The instant the child wakes up pleased and contented, give her a cheerful but firm so-called information jingle x 4, which will both inform and remind her that it is still night and that she should continue to sleep soundly.

At other times during the night, you should not intervene just because the child wakes up and lies in her crib 'talking' for a while. Only calm her if and when she really asks for help. During the hour of the wolf, however, you can jingle preventively *before* she asks for help, but only once.

If, contrary to expectations, she dissolves into despair, and I mean *despair*, you have fanning to fall back on if there's a real emergency. Reposition her firmly and apply the fan silently. Let it take as long as it takes until the little body is heavy with sleep. But only do it once (followed by a jingle that is merged with the confirmation which you give on your way out and from outside the door).

Once you have given this single, confident message that *at night nothing happens*, distract yourself with other sounds and activities around the house so that your ears are not drawn to the threshold of the child's room – and just leave her in peace.

For the child, these sounds, which have nothing to do with her, signify that you are guarding the fort and keeping the wolf at bay. In the child's world, the injunction '*at night we sleep*' does not apply to the guard on night duty!

The *Good-Night's-Sleep Cure* Light

Are fixed routines during the day that important? Our little Lewis, four months, 'leads' us. I am home with him and I love it. Can't you just administer the cure at night?

A schedule facilitates things tremendously. It might not seem so at the beginning, and you could be forgiven for thinking that a strict timetable complicates rather than simplifies life. But when all the pennies drop, both for you and your child, you will see how much time you have over for yourself and how much your child benefits from being able to predict his day. He's not much different from the rest of humanity in that regard!

In the end, your child will become his own clock and will function dependably everywhere. You will be able to plan your days – and evenings – because you will have a freedom of movement that has been inconceivable for many months.

For example, you will be able to devote yourself whole-heartedly to your child when he is awake, since you will know when he is going to go to sleep and for how long. As a result, everything will be so much simpler and so much more fun.

Just the fact that your child will be eating with a hearty appetite will make life far easier.

The fixed routines have more than practical significance. For your child, they mean *security* (see the chapter *Security*), which is of paramount importance.

Carefully thought through, solid routines during the day are the prerequisite for dependable routines at night.

Comforting sick children
Shouldn't you pick up young children when they are sick or having teething problems?

Nothing will improve if the child doesn't sleep.

Think about how you feel when you are sick. Would you want to lie in someone's arms in a bed other than your own if you were burning up with fever? Would you want to get up to be hugged by a bunch of anxious people, eat in the middle of the night, watch TV and socialize? Probably you would want to sleep your way back to health. You would no doubt appreciate it if someone changed your sheets, aired out the room and gave you something to drink, but apart from that, I think you would prefer to be left in peace.

Help your child to sleep!

An unhappy, sick little kid can be comforted in her bed. You can bend down and hold her. You can give her water, cool her down with a compress and calm her. If you are trying to help, you will do a better job if you help on the child's terms and take into account the child's needs rather than focusing on your own.

So comfort and calm a child where she is lying – in her bed, not out of it!

Young children who sleep well and sufficiently long will take teething problems in their stride. Getting a tooth is *not* the same as getting sick or running a fever. That is a myth.

On the other hand, it itches like crazy, so she will probably need a piece of unsweetened crisp bread to gnaw on between meals during the day!

What are we doing wrong?

Things went so well to begin with. The cure was working brilliantly. Heather, eight months, was sleeping longer and longer every night. But now, after nine nights, we seem to be back to square one. She wakes up every other hour and cries so much we have to buff. What are we doing wrong?

She may have had a relapse – rather like dieters who start out strong and lose 15 pounds only to suddenly fall off the wagon and devour an entire cake. It is as though young children need to dive one last time into the dark waters of how things used to be before than can say farewell to all that misery once and for all, find the peace they need and embark upon a new and better life.

Relapses usually pass in one (admittedly horrid) night if the conscientious parents can keep the peace, avail themselves of the strategies the Tool Box has to offer and cultivate that *attitude of supreme confidence.*

The other possibility is that you and your partner may have gotten stuck in a rut. You convey the message endlessly, even though Heather knows perfectly well what's what. You must understand that you are *disturbing* her every time you intervene unnecessarily. Most, if not all, interventions at this stage are not only unnecessary, but are actually acts of sabotage.

Have a little more faith in your daughter! And a little more faith in yourselves!

Stop buffing. You should have said goodbye to all that a long time ago. If there is a real crisis, if she has been lying awake for an eternity and a vicious cycle must be broken, you have fanning to fall back on. However, you should be able to still her crying with the jingle. Intestinal fortitude is what's needed here!

Her confused questions – and this anxious confusion is virtually guaranteed if you bombard her with your own anxiety, which is what you are doing – must have reassuring answers in the form of a loud 'ka-pow!' jingle that terminates the proceedings and unequivocally informs her that she can sleep in peace.

At night nothing happens. The wolf isn't coming. There is no entertainment on offer either. So knock it off! Limit communication traffic – that includes the jingle – to a minimum.

And calm down. Bear in mind that it is appallingly burdensome for a young child to be constantly at the center of attention, perpetually exposed to her parents' over-concentration.

Imagine how you would feel if you were in a restaurant trying to enjoy a fabulous gourmet dinner, while right across the table from you sat someone who didn't eat but just stared at you anxiously the whole time.

'Does it taste good? Is the beef too rare? Too well done? Too cold? Too hot? Would you rather have gone somewhere else? How is the sauce? How are the potatoes? Would you have preferred mashed? Do you want more jelly? How is the salad? You can eat onions, can't you? What if you're allergic? Are you sure you're not allergic? Oh, I'm really worried now. What if you *are* allergic? Are you full now? Do you want some more? Was it too much? Can you eat any more? Did you get enough? Is your stomach upset? Do you want to go to the washroom? And how is the wine? Mellow enough? Too warm? Is it good? Do you want a different wine? Shall I ask for the wine list? Don't you like it? Maybe we could go to another restaurant. Do you want to? We can if you like. *Do* you want to go to another restaurant?'

You would eventually yell at the top of your lungs in front of everyone, 'For God's sake, GET OUT OF MY FACE! Let me eat in peace!'

Young children want to sleep in peace too.

You must realize that it is not just Heather that must take the path to enlightenment. You have to take it too, and you have to do it *first.* You have to step back. You have to chase away the wolves that you have allowed to get right up to Heather's bed side.

Leave, take the wolves with you and shoot them. Learn to have faith in your child and show her respect. Let her enjoy her gourmet sleep and stand guard outside, *away* from her!

Your job is to *guarantee* your child's sleep, not disturb it.

Standing up in bed

I don't even have time to get out of the room before Alexander, 10 months, stands up in his crib and starts to scream bloody murder. It doesn't matter how many times I put him down. He is on his feet again in the blink of an eye.

Little angels who are forever leaping to their feet – let them stand there! Monitor as usual.

If he is angry, ticked off and generally protesting, there is not much to be done, and you shouldn't try. There is no law against standing up, especially if he can lie down again by himself (and he can if no one else is doing it for him).

Nor is there a law against reacting. Quite the contrary, protesting is perfectly benign. An angry little kid has to get his discontent out of his system.

There is, however, a law against becoming really unhappy. At this point, the child is asking for help, and it is only when a child asks for help that he is capable of accepting it.

So, reposition if things get to this stage, but not before. Jingle on the way out and jingle from outside the door. This jingle will be merged with the confirmation jingle and will constitute the last word.

If and when little Alexander has really asked for help, he will stay lying down.

Overworked

My husband took the first two nights, and this evening it was my turn. I had perfected my buffing technique and I used it on Thomas, five months, when I had positioned him in his bed. 'What are you doing?' my husband hissed. 'He's not crying!' I hadn't thought of that...

Well, it's a question of rolling with the punches. The *Good-Night's-Sleep Cure* is a process and little Thomas has already come a long way towards *enjoyment!* (See the chapter of the same title.)

The most common error people make is 'getting stuck'. Don't fall into that trap! When the child cries, both of you should feel as though he is waving you *away* from him rather than *towards* him. You might come to him, if you really think it is necessary, but only to depart again immediately. Every time you get stuck in that proverbial rut and hang around, the wolf sticks his slavering jaws through the door. Then you are the one who is posing the danger to public safety. Think about that!

Your job is to keep the wolf at bay in the space between the locked front door and your child. In other words, the battle takes place outside, not inside the child's room. If the battle is waged from inside the child's room, the child thinks that both of you risk falling victim to the wolf. If no one is standing guard, what will become of us? You are the survival guarantee!

Regular beds
We have set up a room for Sally, two years old. Can we cure her in a regular bed?

Keep the crib (or bring it back)! Two-year-olds are too small to lie in such a vast bed. They will leave it, not so much because they long for the parental bed but because a regular bed has no walls and is therefore not much of a home.

Go back to the good old crib, which used to be Sally's 'room'! Don't introduce the beds with the wide open spaces until after the terrible two's (three and a half to four years old).

The night wanderer

How on earth can I cure John, five years old, who is forever getting out of bed and padding around the house to check out what's going on? When we wake up, we find him in our bed, on the sofa, or in front of the TV(!), but never in his own bed.

People between three and six should not be allowed out of bed. They can lie in the dark and be bored, but they should not get up. Remove any and all interesting objects that happen to be within reach of the bed and of course all lamps. No entertainment. Silence must reign when you are curing night wanderers!

Put him down in good time for a twelve-hour sleep. (Don't forget the bedtime laugh.) Fan in his favorite position with a little pressure to conclude, and then leave the room with a friendly but firm jingle x 4.

Sit with your back to the child on a chair outside the door so that you are in plain view from the child's bed. Busy yourself intently with a silent activity that has nothing to do with little John. Read a book, write a letter, knit, do anything you like as long as whatever it is demands your full attention. Don't look in John's direction. But listen. If he so much as twitches, reply with a gruff jingle that brooks no opposition. If he has time to get up, he won't have time to get out of the room. Grab the little optimist immediately, lead him back to bed and let him scramble under the covers himself, a little pressure over the body, and out with a jingle. Then sit down again and go back to your work. You can leave your post every now and again, but your ears stay put, if you get what I mean!

Stand guard for one night, preferably two. (*Don't* bed down on a mattress on the floor. That's world class entertainment.)

And don't get drawn into a discussion. It's the jingle, and only the jingle, that counts. It says it all.

The cure for night wanderers usually takes three or four nights. If your little wanderer starts to make his rounds after you have gone to bed and fallen asleep, it's a question of popping up before the little angel has had time to pop down and purposefully leading him back to bed and letting him get into the bed himself. No comments. Just wait matter-of-factly until he has gotten himself into bed properly, and then leave immediately with a jingle.

If you are afraid of missing him (with good reason no doubt), when you can't keep your eyes open any longer, there is a technical miracle that is of tremendous help if you have a little night wanderer to deal with – a cordless infrared alarm. Install it close to the bed. It will alert everyone in the house, the wanderer included, that a walkabout is at hand – which should be interrupted immediately as per the instructions above.

Hysteria

What is the difference between your method and the Five-Minute Method? Our little Catherine always got the breast when she got whiny. We thought we would cure her and tried to buff her, but she started to cry hysterically!

Many parents of infants have never heard their children cry. They simply shove in either breast or pacifier the second the baby opens her mouth. Consequently, they think that crying, which should be regarded as either a question or a reaction (with hundreds of variations), is the same as hysteria. It isn't. Hysterical children cry until they vomit, or faint, or both.

Questions in the form of crying (how else can the child express them?) are not indicative of hysteria. They are questions that demand answers that *the child finds satisfactory*. And you mustn't give up until you have succeeded in providing them. It is the child's final *reaction of relief* that tells you that you have hit the mark.

So I don't think that little Catherine is hysterical, and you should be careful about misusing the word hysteria. Hysteria is the manifestation of an unbearable mental state in a child (and in the rest of us for that matter).

In a nutshell, the difference between the Five-Minute Method or the Controlled Crying Method, where the adults are completely passive apart from making an appearance every five minutes, and the *Good-Night's-Sleep Cure*, where the adults both through their words and their actions help the child find peace, is this:

210

- The *Good-Night's-Sleep Cure* requires that the adults take full responsibility for ensuring that their child sleeps well.
- The Five-Minute Method places responsibility for going to sleep and staying asleep on the child.

The reaction to the Five-Minute Method's spineless betrayal, if you will pardon the expression, is, more often than not, (genuine) hysteria.

Uncomfortable clothes

The cure went off without a hitch, but I am having problems with outdoor naps. Alfred, six months, wants to sleep on his stomach in the carriage as well. But he doesn't lie particularly comfortably in his winter overalls. It looks as though he feels a bit cramped. If I try to put him down on his back, he protests by arching his whole body like a bow.

Constricting overalls are not ideal for tummy sleepers who nap out of doors. Think about it. How would you like to be dressed if you had to sleep on a park bench in cold weather? You would certainly want something warm under you and something warm over you as well. But would you be comfortable in thermal pants and a padded overcoat? Dry, thin clothes layer upon layer would be a better solution, don't you think?

It is easy to forget in the fashion obsessed world we live in that clothes should be designed for children, not the other way around!

Better before

We are into the third day of the cure with our little Lily, ten months. Before we made up our schedule and began the cure, she was in the habit of sleeping like a dream at midday. Now the midday nap is the main problem! She refuses to sleep. We don't know what to believe.

Never look back. Don't focus on what used to work and doesn't now, but rather on what was hopeless before and is now beginning to come together. Remember that you can't evaluate anything until you have seen the whole cure through to the end, including the follow-up week.

Young children don't do anything *habitually*. They just do what we teach them. They have their own personalities and their own rhythms, but they are not born with habits and behavior patterns. It is the adults in their lives, us in other words, who decide what their habits, good and bad, are going to be, and children assume that that's the natural order of things. They follow our cues in the belief that we know what we are doing, since we obviously have the ability to navigate our way through this world. We survive and they wonder how we do it.

So don't think in terms of *refuse, don't want to* or even *want to*. Your task is to break a pattern that has become unbearable for all concerned and has utterly exhausted your child. It was easy to teach your child a pattern that brought her distress, and it is just as easy to introduce her to a new pattern. But you have to allow time for all the pennies to drop. Four days and nights plus a follow-up week is hardly an eternity compared to the last nine months, is it?

Re-Cure

I have a confession to make. Slowly but (very) surely we have allowed Gabriel's sleep to go to hell in a hand basket. He is ten months old now.

You must have come across this kind of thing before. It begins with 'It's not a big a deal if he fell asleep with his bottle this evening, is it?' and, after many months of slowly being weaned off the Good-Night's-Sleep Cure, *it ends with having to get up (as we did last night) and 'rock' the crib – we have those bow-shaped attachments on the legs – at least fifteen times (yes, I do hate myself) and still the kid doesn't fall asleep! I'm not exaggerating.*

Naturally we have come to the conclusion that the time has come to deal with this once and for all, but I need your help. On top of everything else, he has a runny nose. Is it really a good idea? (Then again, what's the alternative?)

And since he has 'forgotten' what a good night's sleep really is and will be absolutely furious, I have to know what I'm supposed to DO if he vomits or faints. And since we are stuck in rocking mode, we have to break that pattern, don't we? And just rely on the jingle?

This certainly isn't the first time I have read a confession like this! I'm surprised, saddened and somewhat irritated when people are careless about preserving something as precious as a sound sleep – but perhaps it was too easy to bring about?!

But of course I understand. There is so much that has to be understood: that young children grow, that they are not newborns forever (and not Cure children forever), that the course has to be re-plotted at regular intervals, just as schedules, menus, wardrobes and everything else has to be adjusted as time passes. You always have to be one step ahead. Where is it all going to lead?

With twenty-twenty hindsight, you will learn to think ahead, and it's little Gabriel who is teaching you. You should thank him for that! It will stand you in good stead throughout his childhood!

So you are trying to rock the crib? That is not particularly effective. You are obviously stuck in a rut, so break out of it. Start by thinking in terms of *out* rather than in. Haven't you started to buff him?

Decide where you want to start! I would go with corrective positioning, kindly but firmly, and then I would buff. Do it just as the *Good-Night's-Sleep Cure* is described in the Cheat Sheet. If he is buffed, he *can't* scream himself into hysteria. It just isn't possible if you have developed a sufficiently effective technique. So vomiting and fainting can be struck from the agenda!

I also might conclude that he does in fact know what the drill is and would stick to fanning after corrective positioning, from the top down, static, steady and long, until his entire little body was heavy with sleep. A final nudge and then out with a jingle. I wouldn't hesitate to stand by his bed side for ten minutes if that's what it took at this stage of the game so that he would be guaranteed enough time to fall silent and be still. If, when I left and began to jingle, he still got angry in spite of everything, that's allowed. See the Cheat Sheet!

If he then really worked himself up to the point where I thought things were getting seriously unpleasant, I would rush in and repeat corrective positioning and fanning. I wouldn't be particularly sweet about it either. I would be clear and firm, although not angry or unkind. And I wouldn't stay ten minutes but two. Then out with a jingle and away from the door with an abridged confirmation.

If, in spite of my assiduous ministrations, he started to sound sad and tired and didn't settle down with the reminder jingle but stubbornly continued to ask for help, he would get it – same procedure but a touch softer, still neither sweet nor comforting mind you, but decisively *reassuring*.

I would count on two tough nights with a lot of running back and forth (although the time you spend running will decrease). Work on the jingle so that it gets through to him unequivocally. It should be nagging and firm so that there is no doubt in his mind that I/the jingle/sleep cannot be negotiated with. I would make up my mind to restore order both in the child and in myself.

And since order once reigned, I would assume that the re-cure would get back into that groove relatively quickly and that the *Good-Night's-Sleep Cure* would therefore go that much faster.

Don't worry about the runny nose. Not sleeping won't make his cold any better.

(Continued) When we administered the cure more than four months ago (which we slowly and steadily dismantled), everything felt wonderful once we were done. But after a while, when we had acclimatized and the problems started, it was so easy to give the 'wrong answers' to his questions – in the beginning all it took was one shake of the crib for him to fall back to sleep... But we SHOULD have jingled and put up with an hour (?) of crying at the most. It's just that at the time that seemed like the toughest alternative at least in the short term.

Short-term solutions work once – but not the time after or the time after that. Children are loud and clear on that point. If you pick up a young child half an hour too early in the morning, the kid will wake up exactly half an hour early the next morning and – presto – you are back to square one. It doesn't take that many nights.

You can do it! But your underlying assumption should not be that he is going to scream but that he is going to be *allowed* (NB!) to sleep.

(Continued) Tonight's the night. We are stocking up on coffee and cookies to take us through the wee small hours when everything is at its darkest. It's going to be fun ha ha! A day like this is not something I would like to experience more than once – hopelessness, powerlessness, despair are only the half of it...

How do you stay a step ahead? Is it just a question of resigning yourself to the fact that he is going to cry at bedtime for example? (It must be, no?) The fact that he is feeling mommy and daddy deprived right now and doesn't want to be alone, does that play in?

Now I must object. You are assuming that he is going to cry. Why? Your task (and your husband's) is to calm him. That is what the strategies described in the cure are for. He won't cry at all! At least not in the way that you mean. He is not going to cry in a way that demands pity. He *is asking questions!* Or, alternatively, reacting to the answers.

The fact that he isn't as happy as he once was is the result of that unpleasant association with the wolf (your anxiety, your insecurity, your mixed messages), and his own sleep deprivation. His sleep deprivation is at least as serious as yours. But all this will pass when he becomes *secure in himself* and is permitted/can/dares to sleep well at night. So you have done him a disservice here. Out with the wolves of anxiety! That's the primary goal!

(Continued) As far as we can make out, your theory that he still knows the drill seems to be right. We had a good laugh last thing before corrective positioning at 8.02. He asked questions persistently until 8.28 – but the jingle only had to be said

twice during this time, and it was close to the end that I gave the confirmation. It was 8.29 when he took the last confirmation with him into dreamland and he is still asleep now (9.04). Normally, we would have been in to rock the bed two or three times by now.

Great! Now I also want to hear that both of you have really assumed your roles as confident leaders so that you don't fall into the trap of thinking that little Gabriel is going to take care of the cure, his sleep, the decisions, the answers, the messages, the nights, the routines, and life itself for the two of you!

(Continued) I beg leave to defend myself! I have in fact understood the Good-Night's-Sleep Cure. What frightens me the most, if I can put it like that, is the fact that we got stuck in almost everything the last time. If it wasn't rocking, it was buffing and then jingling. Whatever we did, we got stuck. It is the knowledge that I have to abruptly stop overusing the tools that has me spooked. I think to myself, 'What do I have left to fall back on?' But I have realized that what I have left is precisely the Good-Night's-Sleep Cure! As it should be administered. No half measures, no maybe's, no what-if's... Just the Good-Night's-Sleep Cure from A to Z, just as you have described it! I'm ashamed to admit that we actually tried to administer the cure without the bedtime laugh. God knows what we thought we were doing...

His answers were obviously so relieved that you didn't have to work very hard (or at all!). Perhaps the jingle never took over the way it was supposed to – so that it alone was sufficient to trigger that conditioned reflex that causes a child to fall asleep or at least lie down so peacefully. Then you began to run in and out to check on things – which you should only do once the child has been asleep for ten minutes. With all your running in and out, you disturbed him and all the through traffic gave rise to anxiety. You let in the wolf. It is like the guard out there on the battle field. He has to gaze into the distance away towards the horizon to discover possible threats. He should not tip toe around among the soldiers who are sleeping, or at least trying to sleep, and stare at them anxiously. They should be able to sleep soundly precisely because he is standing guard! That's the whole point of the exercise!

If you don't understand *why* the *Good-Night's-Sleep Cure* works, you are easy prey for doubt when you are trying to understand *how* it works and put it into practice.

(Continued) Just have to quickly tell you that right now – quarter to eight in the morning – he is sleeping so beautifully. There are not going to be any problems. I can feel it. Of course he woke up and howled with outrage ten times before midnight, but then not a sound! And the longest bout only lasted 12 minutes. And how long is that really? And he 'demanded' not even one jingle after he fell asleep! The question is how the jingle can produce a conditioned reflex if we never have to use it. He fixes it himself in the end.

I am very, very happy today, and I think Gabriel will be too when his dad wakes him up at eight o'clock!

Well done! Not even any problems during the hour of the wolf. Everything will settle very soon when the pre-midnight complaining begins to die away, which will happen as early as tonight.

Try to make sure that the jingle always has the last word as a confirmation so that he takes it with him when he falls asleep. (That means every time he wakes up and *asks questions* in the form of crying, not when he comes to and merely talks a little, and falls back to sleep by himself.)

(Continued) Last night went brilliantly! He asked questions for eight minutes when he was put down and then woke up twice after one hour but was only awake for a minute both times. Then he slept until we woke him! On the other hand, when he went down for the first daytime nap, he cried for eight minutes again and then slept for 35 minutes. Then we had to jingle a little and reposition once, since he was really ticked off and very unhappy right up to when we picked him up fifteen minutes before his time. He was supposed to sleep for one and a half hours. So he 'cried' for 45 minutes... And right now, an hour and fifteen minutes later, he is really

tired. And he has a bad cold on top of everything else. You can imagine what kind of a mood he is in. And his next nap isn't for another three hours... I know we had problems with the daytime naps last time too. He would wake up too early and never go back to sleep. So we decided he could take a 45-minute nap instead of the one-and-a-half-hour version on the days this happened. Letting the naps change places – that's the wrong way to go, isn't it?

Great! What a night! Full marks!

But you have to cure according to the rules during the days as well. Everything is connected to everything else. Thinking in terms of compensation is a betrayal. It may seem like a good idea at the time, but it inevitably leads to confusion. So keep to the schedule! Frame it and put it up on the wall. Give him the prerequisites and assume that he will put them to good use (eventually)! And remember that you can always splice in a brief nap of (exactly) five minutes (on the child's initiative) if there is a crisis without compromising the schedule.

(Continued) Everything is going well for the most part. At bedtime he asks questions for about eight minutes. It's worse during the days. It can take up to 20 minutes before he goes to sleep. But at least he goes to sleep by himself! I am really happy about that. And we hardly ever need to jingle. He's mostly angry, never sad.

On the other hand, I am having serious problems getting the humorless little gangster to laugh. He isn't even ticklish! He starts to cry angrily as soon as we come into the room and he realizes that it is bed time. From what I understand, it's not supposed to be this way. What do you think?

Good that he is angry. That is allowed. Just cultivate the jingle, I beg you! The jingle is your best friend, a companion you always want by your side. Use it! Send a confirmation with him into dreamland, no matter how ticked off he is. It will pass.

He won't even let himself be tickled? What a sad sack! But, like all kids, he needs some fun in his life. Experiment! Clown around. Play peek-a-boo, 'fall', trip, tickle his loving dad (that would be fun, wouldn't it? You're too tired? You're kidding!). Turn him around (the kid, not the dad), lift him up and down, and let him look at himself in the mirror. You and your husband can joke around with each other and roar with laughter. Use your imagination! Angry crying you just don't hear. Concentrate on each other and put Gabriel to bed as though it's an afterthought. Go on fooling around without paying him much attention or any attention at all until he *wants* to laugh (and he will). He is more than welcome to think that you are both off your rockers as long as he gets bored with being angry and sulky. Sooner or later it is going to happen!

(To conclude) Two weeks have gone by since I first wrote to you, and Gabriel is sleeping just the way he should from eight at night to eight in the morning. Yesterday evening it was three (!!!) minutes before he got a confirmation and he accepted it without a word!

During the day, it takes him four to five minutes to fall asleep, but then he sleeps right up until he is supposed to wake up. And he is so happy and perky during the day – and one tough little trooper too. He took his first steps a week ago!

Now we are all sleeping well. I had forgotten how glorious it was...

Curing twins

Can we cure our twins, five months, together? Both kids are sleeping in the parental bed, since the two little gangsters rejected cribs from day one. Their mother (me) lies in bed like a rotating milk machine rolling from one side of the bed to the other and feeding them both all night. If the truth be told, I am yearning for the day when I can both go to sleep and wake up with my dear husband by my side. How can I apply your cure on these two? Is there some kind of spell we can cast to make them both fall asleep at the same time? Or should we start by curing one of them and, once he has learned to fall asleep by himself, let the other follow in his brother's footsteps?

Cure them both at once! You will be jumping from crib to crib like a flea on a hot brick – especially on the first night before the jingle takes over – and that's no picnic, but I've done it a couple of times and it *is* possible. There are two of you after all (I was alone!) and you and your husband can take a kid each. Cure them both at the same time. Lose the pacifiers (if any) – they only complicate things. Draw up a schedule with a twelve-hour night (or eleven if it suits you better) as per the instructions in the Tool Box and make the appropriate preparations. It is all laid out for you. They can sleep in the same room but they should not be able to see each other if and when they wake up.

(To conclude) I just wanted to write and tell you that we have a cheery and contented set of twins in the house, who sleep like logs the whole night through in their own beds! The cure has succeeded beyond our wildest dreams, even though we had a couple of trying nights. Now the little rascals sleep eleven hours from eight at night until seven the next morning. I can sometimes hear that they are awake, but they are not unhappy and fall back to sleep very quickly. Fantastic!

Evening crying
Our daughter, who is four months old, starts to cry as soon as she is put down in the carriage for the night. This has been going on since the first day of the cure, and she is a very unhappy little girl. I rock her immediately, since it doesn't take her long to 'rev up'. What am I doing wrong? Why does she cry? This happens so rarely during the day. I just put her down when she is still awake. She wriggles around for a little while but then goes to sleep.

The problem is your negative expectations! You rock her immediately in the evening because you know that it doesn't take long for her to 'rev up'. How do you know that? I think it is your negative expectations that she is defending herself against. She is simply sad because you make going to bed in the evenings so hard for her, instead of making it as simple and self-evident as it is during the day. Negative expectations are just as self-fulfilling as positive ones.

So stop rocking. Reposition her, push the carriage back and forth a couple of times and then *leave* and, from a safe distance, give her a jingle x 4.

I also suspect that she needs a bedtime top up. Your breasts are a little tired in the evenings. There's not much milk left and the little that does remain is on the thin side. You need a supplement! At four months, she also needs something besides breast milk during the day.

You are not forgetting the bedtime laugh, are you?

So tired

Is it normal for a child to be extra tired during the cure? My little boy Erik, four months, is so tired and whiny during the day. Should I let him sleep more than 15–16 hours out of 24, or will I ruin his night sleep if I let him sleep more during the day?

Yes, it is normal. The more he sleeps, the more tired – and the sleepier – he will get during the cure. He has a lot of catching up to do. The tide will turn when it turns. And it *will* turn, never fear.

Don't play around with your carefully thought out schedule! You can't really evaluate it until after the follow-up week. Stick to the timetable, even thought it's tough at times. Doing anything else is less than kind to little Erik.

In emergencies, you always have a margin of 5, 10 or 15 minutes (never more).

To bed a couple of hours later?

Our son Linus is five months old. We were wondering if once he is sleeping according to the schedule, are we locked into that particular timetable forever, or can we put him to bed a couple of hours later if, for example we have been asked out for the evening?

The timetable transforms the child into his own clock. After the cure – and you should count on it taking upwards of a month before everything has really settled down – you will be able to take little Linus with you anywhere, put him to bed anywhere, take him home and put him back down in his own bed to go on sleeping without disturbing him in the least. Anyone will be able to put him to bed anywhere, just as anyone will be able to feed him anywhere – with the proviso that everyone concerned *sticks to the timetable.*

Messing with the timetable is risky. We adults can stay up until four in the morning the odd night if there's a party. We know what it will cost us in terms of lost sleep, fatigue and perhaps a hangover. We choose to pay the price, but young children can't choose. Their fate is entirely in our hands. For a child that young 'a couple of hours later' is major jet lag!

So I don't see why a child's timetable shouldn't be accorded the same respect as an adult's.

Starving?

Our twin girls are six months old. We want to cure them. At the moment, the day starts around seven, but since they are still eating during the night, they are not hungry until eight. Won't it throw the timetable off a bit if they are hungrier early in the morning and want to eat as soon as they wake up? Can they really get through a whole night without food? Do kids that have been cured usually wake up ravenous?

No. The great thing is that cutting out the night feeding influences *the day,* not the morning. You will be surprised over their lack of interest in food after a twelve-hour fast. They will only start eating more heartily on the third day of the cure and not until the fourth, fifth or sixth day will they start eating as they should in the morning. They no longer need a night feeding, and I can guarantee that they won't starve to death!

(Continued) Do we have to stick rigidly to the schedule even though everything has solidified and runs like clockwork? Will we ruin everything when we go to stay with my parents in a little over two weeks?

Once all the pennies have dropped and everything has settled down, you will see what a blessing hard and fast routines are and how much freedom of movement they give you. You will be the schedule's staunchest defender!

Traveling is no problem, but stick to the schedule I implore you! A lot of people think that when they go away on a trip they can cast the schedule to the four winds and reintroduce it when they get home. That's not the way it works unfortunately. As far as kids are concerned, there is not a whole lot of difference between a trip and a move. They will happily reorient themselves when they get home, but they may be a touch surprised since they thought they had moved on with you. So stick to the schedule and let the kids take it with them wherever they go! You will avoid a whole slew of problems.

An active child
My partner and I have decided that our daughter Nicole, seven months, should start sleeping through the nights. It's not going that well. We think that she should be dog tired, since she sleeps so little during the day. She takes a 30-minute nap in the morning and sleeps a maximum of 45 minutes in the afternoon. She is, and always has been, a really active kid.

Illogical though it might sound, the less she sleeps during the day, the worse she will sleep at night. Thus, skimping on the naps in the belief that she will sleep longer at night will get you nowhere. If she gets too little sleep during the day, all that will happen is that she will get overtired. And she will have as much trouble finding peace as an overtired adult would.

You should also know that the overwhelming majority of children are incredibly active. They just keep going until they literally collapse. They are programmed to develop at breakneck speed. It's almost as though someone is cracking a whip over their heads. You are hardly doing Nicole a favor by not helping her find the peace she so desperately needs.

Little Nicole needs approximately 14.5 hours of sleep out of every 24.

Howling... but no more

We are desperate for advice on how to help our little son Jason to sleep soundly. He is now seven months old and he has great difficulty sleeping at night. I got onto your web page and read the Cheat Sheet for the Good-Night's-Sleep Cure. We did our best to follow the instructions. We drew up a schedule and so on. All that happened was he screamed his head off until he suddenly passed out. In other words, the part of the process when you say the jingle before leaving was really problematic. He would immediately start to howl and would pull himself up.

We are really trying hard to teach him to fall asleep to the jingle, but more often than not he screams even louder when we say it. It seems as though he associates the jingle with screaming rather than sleeping. Getting him to fall asleep always involves at least half an hour of screaming both day and night, and I feel very badly about that. I don't know where to turn!

You haven't gotten the hang of buffing him until he is calm and quiet. You and your partner should practice on each other. You should also prepare yourselves mentally, which I don't think you have done either. The attitude of supreme confidence is the key. I strongly recommend the chapters entitled *Peace* and *Security*.

You have also gotten stuck on saying the jingle in the room, where it won't do any good. Quite the contrary, it opens the door for the wolf. So read, read and practice hard! What you are supposed to do and why is outlined in the Cheat Sheet and the Tool Box. There is also a description of what the jingle elicits in the beginning, namely renewed questions, and how important an answer the jingle is.

(Continued) Jason is now sleeping continuously from 7.00 at night until 6.30 in the morning! The transformation he has gone through is quite extraordinary, and it is fascinating to see how effective the jingle is now. If he wakes up during the night, all we have to do is say it, and he is off back to sleep immediately.

It can still be a problem to get him to fall asleep peacefully in the evening. He is always unhappy for a while before he settles, but even this has begun to improve.

Wonderful! Preserve all the good results you have achieved thus far, and stick to the schedule! *If you don't call your child's sound night sleep into question, neither will he.*

Never neglect the bed time laugh! The more fun he has and the more he laughs before he goes down for the night (a procedure that should take two minutes at the most), the closer he gets to *enjoyment* and the faster everything will go. If you take no notice of his little breakdown, after all the fun you both have had, and simply leave the room with a happy, spirited almost brisk jingle, he will soon grow weary of feeling sorry for himself... and realize that falling into a contented sleep is a lot more fun and a lot more comfortable.

Remember to say good morning with great fanfare too! A new day should be greeted just as joyously as a comfortable night.

(To conclude) We are now into our seventh night and Jason is sleeping right through without even waking up once. The last two nights, even the bedding procedure has been going smoothly and has only taken about five minutes, which really feels good. If you only knew how much the whole family fools around and laughs in the evening! I feel so exhilarated and happy afterwards.

I am really fascinated by the fact that all this is even possible. It makes me believe that we can achieve anything if we just put our minds to it.

A big thank you for all your help and support. We have done a lot more than just teach Jason to sleep well. My husband and I now feel far more secure as parents because we were able to face the problem and together succeed in breaking an unhealthy pattern.

Cure

Marisa is eight months old. You write that children of five to six months should be sleeping twelve-hour nights. That seems so unattainable to us. My husband and I had tried everything (at least we thought we had) until I read about the Good-Night's-Sleep Cure. *This is our last hope. We really need your help!*

You can put up with sleep deprivation for five to six months. Then the parents start to unravel, not to mention the child. If it continues, everyone involved usually crashes and burns when the child is eight to nine months old. I think you should administer the *Good-Night's-Sleep Cure* exactly as it is laid out. No sidesteps! The results you want are not at all unattainable. They are ready and waiting for you just around the corner! Little Marisa is made of exactly the same stuff as all young children (and everyone else): flesh and blood. Her needs are as common to the rest of humanity as yours are.

(Continued) We have been gearing up and preparing each other for Friday, when we plan to start the Good-Night's-Sleep Cure. *We have a question before we take the plunge. It's about the 'jingle'. Should the jingle always be the same, or does it vary depending on the message? The reminder for example?*

Same jingle, different tone of voice. Practice – preferably a long way from home so you don't scare the neighbors... It can be high or low, tender or decisive. The variations are endless, but think opera! The jingle should rise from your gut and be said with force. You can choose among jingle x 4, x 6 or even x 8 on occasion. You will develop a knack for hearing her 'answers' and knowing when you have to reel off one or two more verses. You will say the verses in one fell swoop without even a hint of hesitation in between. Read about this in the Tool Box.

(Continued) Report on day 1:
We got through the first night and it went very well! We were prepared for catastrophe, but it was a walk in the park. Incredible. No breastfeeding no endless walking with the child in my arms. She hardly woke up at all and slept for long periods. Will we run into problems tonight?
When she sleeps in the carriage, is it OK to push it around or should the carriage be stationary?

There won't be any problems at all. Quite the contrary, you will go from success to success!

Pushing the carriage around is fine when you're out, but park it too so she sleeps while it's not moving. She should get used to both. Rock her forcefully to send a message if she wakes up early and then park the carriage for a while so she has time to fall back to sleep properly before you continue your walk. *(Continued) In preparation for the second night, we have followed the daytime schedule slavishly. We put her down at 7.00 p.m. and she was asleep by 7.08!*

Questions: After leaving the room how long should we let Marisa cry before we do something about it? How long should she be silent before we give her the confirmation?

Impossible to say. It's not a matter of time, but *how* she cries. Is she angry? Surly? Is she feeling sorry for herself? Is it a reaction? A question? A protest? Is she really unhappy?

In the last case, she should be given a reminder fairly promptly. It should be reassuring, soothing and loud. The rest of the procedure will take as long as it takes. See The Cheat Sheet: *Monitor.* Give her time and listen long and carefully. Mentally, where is she going? 'Down?' Wait and splice in a confirmation jingle when she starts to quiet down. You are better off being too early than too late, so she has time to fall asleep. She might get her second wind and start up again – whereupon you deliver the reminder again, wait and then finally deliver the confirmation as soon as you hear that she is headed in the right direction. The calm confirmation of the all-is-well variety is what Marisa should take with her as she drifts off to sleep.

(Continued) Report on day 2:
This night went even better! By 11.00 p.m., Marisa had woken up five times (one round of buffing and one of corrective positioning). After that, she woke up only once (!) at 5.27 a.m., and my husband jingled from outside the door. She quieted right down and went back to sleep. Incredible! I'm the point person the next two nights, so we'll see if she reacts differently.

Congratulations! So tonight is your turn. That can cause a little confusion at the beginning (less so the next night). Now it is extra important that you put Marisa to bed with great fanfare and much laughter (before Dad disappears). You will confirm each other, and Marisa won't have to wonder whether Dad's on board with everything or whether the wolf is going to show up now that Mom is 'alone' in the world... Same procedure in the morning. Both of you are there to strike up the band! That will also serve to confirm that all is right with the world and that all three of you are a team.

(Continued) Unfortunately, Marisa hasn't quite twigged to the fact that Mom is the one who is in charge of the bedding procedure now. I was putting her down for her afternoon nap (12.30 to 2.00), and there were wild protests! Are setbacks like this normal when the mother takes over?

New questions – not setbacks – are normal when parent number two takes the wheel. Nothing wrong with that. The child is in the process of figuring out the rules of the game. Nip confusion in the bud by conducting yourself in an indefatigably reassuring manner without so much as a whisper of hesitation.

(Continued) I am so happy with how the night went! We have really been communicating and it's so fabulous! I have so much more confidence in myself and I feel more secure when I jingle.

Great! The next step is to get her to fall asleep by herself, so tonight you will wait even longer before you deliver the reminder, and you will listen long and hard to ascertain what headspace she is occupying. When you feel a dialogue starting, merge the reminder and the confirmation. You will jingle x 6 (or even x 8) in one shot. Be a little softer towards the end when you hear that she is beginning to answer and settle down during the reminder. Now she is beginning to understand the drill and is becoming more secure in herself. You are doing a sterling job!
(Continued) Report on day 4

What happened last night was... absolutely nothing! Marisa slept the whole night from 7.00 in the evening until seven the next morning!!! She woke up twice but went back to sleep before I even had time to get to the door.

I think she is already happier and more alert, more into playing with her toys, more curious etcetera!

Now development will literally explode. She will become stronger and happier with each day that passes! But she will be sleepier and more tired for a little while, now that she can finally sleep. Any residual sleep deprivation will manifest itself during the day (and 'latent' cramps can flare up too, now that she has the strength to cope with them). And a relapse may occur – but only for *one* night – so don't get worried. Just use the tools available to you in the *Good-Night's-Sleep Cure* stubbornly – and sparingly. As far as I can make out, however, it's plain sailing from here on in. If you don't call Marisa's night sleep into question, she certainly won't.

Over onto his back
Harry, six months old, has started going to sleep on his back occasionally. Should we try and turn him over, or will he sleep just as well on his back?

The fact that he turns over and lies on his back means nothing. What is important is *that* he sleeps, not *how*. To make sure he sleeps longer, you can always turn him over when he has been asleep for ten minutes (not 20). He won't notice. It's enough to take him by the arm or hand, and gently and careful flip him. Harry will 'believe' that he has turned over by himself and will soon start doing it of his own accord.

The five minute nap
We began the Good-Night's-Sleep Cure *yesterday evening. One question that came up had to do with the daytime schedule. It seems as though we are going to*

have to squeeze in an afternoon nap, since little Mimi, nine months, doesn't seem to be able to stay awake for that five-hour stretch. Do you have any suggestions, or should we wait and see, and try to keep her awake?

When young children suddenly are allowed to sleep through the night, they react with overwhelming fatigue, which they can 'afford' to feel just because they now sleep more. It is way too early to evaluate the situation. You always have the five-minute nap up your sleeve, which you can help her take any time, any place – preferably somewhere at the center of the action. Help her get started by buffing a little. The five-minute snooze is a little power nap that you can let Mimi enjoy outside the schedule without throwing anything out of sync. But check the clock. Five minutes is your window, not a second more or less. When you wake her up, you will have a brand new baby! (Except perhaps the first time, when she will certainly protest and want to sleep longer.)

Cure with impediments
Yesterday evening was the opening salvo of the Good-Night's-Sleep Cure *for Richard, ten months. I am taking all the night shifts, since I think his dad is too 'kind'. Sure enough he got up in the middle of the night when Richard had been crying for a while and felt sorry for him. I was able to shoo him away. If I hadn't, I doubt Richard would have been allowed to stay where he was... Is it OK if I am in charge of all the nights during the cure, even though Dad will take over later? I'm not sure he can handle this, even though he is a really fabulous father!*

Absolutely. As long as someone spells you during the day so that you can sleep, just go on doing what you're doing. And from the third night on, you will be able to grab a reasonably long nap every now and then. The loving father can always get in on the act later. You will soon feel that you are on top of things, and then he can take over with you as his coach. See the cure through as thoroughly as you can. That's what's important. It requires time and a stalwart woman!

Report on day 2:
Today we are fit as fiddles. Richard grumbled a little at 1.30 a.m. and fell back to sleep on two jingles. It didn't take more than a minute! Then all was quiet until 6.20. I can't believe it! I'm just waiting for the big backlash later on in the week...

Super! Wait for the big backlash if you like... It may come, but it won't be a problem because you know what to do and what not to do. (Focus on the latter!) What's important, if and when the backlash comes, is to keep your composure i.e. that attitude of supreme confidence which doesn't permit even the smallest wolf to creep over the threshold and threaten you or little Richard!

Report on day 3:
The metamorphosis that you predicted for the third day has not materialized. On the contrary, Richard is unusually whiny today.

He won't get perkier for a while yet. On the contrary, he will be sleepy for the next little while, instead of being constantly tired. But his appetite will be better and he'll get some roses in his cheeks!

(Continued) Now something has happened that wasn't supposed to happen. Richard has a fever. No other symptoms yet, but he is clingy (for reasons we now know) and is hardly eating at all. How shall I tackle this? I have read that you shouldn't pick children up if they are sick, but isn't it mega bad luck that this had to happen during the cure? I am wondering how I am going to keep going with this – and whether I even ought to! How am I going to cope with his increasing need for sleep during the day for example? And what am I supposed to do if he needs water at night?

Richard has been able to sleep much better than before, and this equips him to cope with illness in a completely different way. He is beginning to develop powers to do battle with things that have been lying latent. You know how adults can get terribly sick as soon as we take a vacation... Yes, it's bad luck, but hardly unusual. So keep going as though nothing has happened, and remember that it is *particularly* important that he get his good night's sleep now that he is sick.

If you think that his forehead feels so hot that giving him water is essential, hold him by his armpits with one arm behind his back/neck and give him water with your free hand in bed. Just get the water into him. Don't fish for approval. If he needs water, he will gratefully accept it, even if he is sleeping. He doesn't need to be sat up or even wake up properly. Try not to disturb him otherwise. He needs to be allowed to sleep his way back to health.

As far as daytime naps go, you have that fifteen minute margin in both directions. Thus, every nap can begin fifteen minutes early and end fifteen minutes late, which means that you can give him an extra half hour every time he needs it without compromising the routines you are in the process of introducing. Fresh air in the room! At night (but only at night), you can also put him to bed a whole half hour earlier without throwing the schedule off, which is good to know.

Report on day 4:
This is how things went: the bedding procedure took two minutes. I guess he was just dead tired, but I thought he seemed to be more aware of things than before! Between 2.00 a.m. and 2.34 a.m., he woke up a few times but went back to sleep on the jingle. I went in and checked his forehead (for fever) after ten minutes, but everything felt OK. That was the last time I was in. He woke up at 7.00 a.m. full of beans. This is the first time that the timetable was adhered to perfectly. I am the happiest person in the world today!

Great job! He has gotten himself a mellow mother. That beats seven Panadol any day!

The left corner

My son Harold, eight months, crawls up to one corner of the crib. I don't know whether he feels shut in (infants like enclosed spaces, don't they?) or he is trying to get out. Crawling up is relatively easy, but crawling back down is an entirely different proposition.

Repositioned him a couple of times, but he got angry.

He also ends up face down on the mattress fairly often. He sleeps for a while, but eventually wants to change position. (No surprise there.) I don't want to go in and disturb him too often. What should I do?

He crawls up to the left-hand corner, right? That is very common! It is just as common for parents to carry their child nestled on their left shoulders.

Young children like a limited world. They are also keen on practicing their crawling (if they get the chance). Wait until he has been asleep for ten minutes. Then you can go in and pull or lift him down without his noticing (and pave the way for him to crawl up again). But don't irritate him by questioning the position he chooses while he is awake!

Face into the mattress is also normal. Don't ask me why it's such a popular pastime... He can lift and turn his head whenever he wants, and this he will do before he goes to sleep.

Time differences

We have cured our little Juliet (13 months) and gotten ourselves a wonderful life! Now we are going to Thailand in October and we will be there for three weeks. There is a six-hour time difference. Can you give me some advice on how to best get her over jet lag on the way out and on the way back?

Make use of that fifteen minute margin. Having their rhythms thrown out of sync *is* a problem for young children, but a quarter of an hour here and there won't make much of an impression and it doesn't compromise the schedule. You can start each point in the program fifteen minutes earlier or fifteen minutes later (depending on whether you are flying east or west). You end up with two or three hours per day in the right direction. You decide how fast you want to make the transition! In your case, the readjustment will take two or three days. With a hard and fast schedule as your foundation and your meticulous attention to duty, tackling the problem of crossing time zones will go very smoothly, and your child's inner clock won't be thrown off.

The following is a tip you didn't ask for, but I will give it to you anyway. Make sure you pack a length of clothes line, some clothes pegs and a couple of black sheets. Being able to shut out the light effectively is invaluable.

Night terror

When our son William, one year old, was seven months, we administered the Good-Night's-Sleep Cure. *And hallelujah! He slept almost twelve hours. But then something happened. Unfortunately, I don't remember what triggered it, whether it was illness or something else... but now we are in a situation where he refuses to go to bed.*

Here's what I was thinking. We have tried countless different methods. Maybe it's time to follow his lead? So the last few nights, we have let him stay up until he falls asleep. Yesterday evening, at around 10.30, I gave up, took him into our bed and breastfed him until he fell asleep. But he still woke up after a while and started to scream. Sleeping beside me doesn't seem to make any difference.

I've heard people talk about something called night terror. We were wondering if that was the problem.

Such a shame that you didn't preserve those good nights but instead started to call them into question! The all important message you must always keep in mind and convey through your attitude is this: *At night we sleep. At night nothing happens.* If you start picking a child up, no matter what the reason, the whole edifice soon collapses. The child becomes anxious and senses danger.

What is called 'night terror', a designation that was coined relatively recently, is what I call The Wolf – or, more accurately, a whole pack of them!

The only solution is to administer the *Good-Night's-Sleep Cure* again – only this time, carefully preserve the results. As you already noticed, following your child's lead doesn't work. He is far too young to even think about shouldering the responsibility for his own sleep routines. The responsibility is yours. So show some leadership and help him! You wouldn't expect him to take responsibility for his mealtimes, would you?

(Continued) We are now on our seventh night, and it's been up and down. Nights three and four were super! William went to sleep with barely a whimper. He only woke up a few times. He whined a little, but went back to sleep almost immediately. On the fifth night, my husband took over. And then things got worse again. I recognize the pattern from the last time. But at least we've made a fresh start and we are doing our best!

One last question: how long should we follow the schedule during the day? Can we expect to be able to improvise a little more eventually?

Improvisations are not advisable for a very, very long time. That would be like trying to teach William how to tell the time and then moving the hands and switching all the numbers on the clock face around. That would hardly make life easier for him!

Fixed times are of decisive importance for young children. (See the chapter entitled *Security*.) It is essential to follow the schedule with a margin of no more than fifteen minutes either way if you want reliably peaceful nights. Soon you will see how hard and fast routines, which enable the child to become his own clock, will simplify your lives beyond belief. Existence becomes predictable for both of you and for William, which will give you all the flexibility you could wish for.

Eat happy
We are just about to embark upon the cure, and my husband and I are wondering if I should stop breastfeeding our ten-month-old daughter Sarah in the evening.

As things stand now, we get her into her pyjamas, draw the curtains, turn off the lights and then she is breastfed (around 7.00 p.m.). She eats and is almost asleep by the time I put her into bed. I now understand that this is a problem. The fact that she almost falls asleep at my breast means that she needs the breast again in order to go on sleeping.

But what shall we do? Should we give her formula instead, or will that lead to the same problem – falling asleep with the bottle? This is a young lady who eats very badly. She has only gained 800 grams in five months. She becomes very restless and bored when she eats unless something interesting is happening. When we are out at a restaurant, she eats a lot, but seldom does so at home.

I think that when she sleeps badly and on top of that is fed during the night, it causes her to lose her appetite during the day. Shall we just skip feeding her at 7.00 in the evening?

Little Sarah needs to have clear boundaries between the various points in the program: either you eat or you sleep and ne'er the twain shall meet. So don't let her doze off at your breast. By all means give her a bedtime top up, but not where she sleeps. Feed her on the sofa with the lights on. Laughing should be the last thing she does, and she should laugh all the way to bed.

Her appetite will improve dramatically when she stops eating at night, but it will take her 72 hours to realize that she is in fact hungry. If you are worried that she isn't getting enough to eat when you breastfeed her in the evening, give her a bottle. Her tummy should be full to bursting, so don't skip the evening top up, whatever you do!

The fact that she eats better when you are out might hinge on little things such as fresh air, your own positive attitude and a spirit of adventure. Nursing isn't always the most exciting activity in the world, especially if you're not very hungry. But her appetite will improve as good sleep patterns are established, along with a well planned schedule with meals at set times and at three-and-a-half-hour intervals.

Pooping during the night

We were wondering how we should proceed when Adrian, nine months, poops during the night.

If little Adrian insists on pooping at night, you will have to learn to change him in his bed! Don't speak, rely on the light from the hall, reposition him when you are done, then a little pressure over his back and out with a jingle. If you pick him up, he will think one of two things: it is morning or the wolf is panting at the door, neither of which is true so we don't want to fib.

Later, when timetables and routines have stabilized, he won't poop at night but rather (my hot tip of the week) at 9.50 in the morning!

Daytime naps in bed

It has become more and more difficult to get little Molly, nine months, to sleep in the carriage despite the fact that our schedule is cast in stone. She is also too big for it now. We were thinking that one of these days we would start putting her down in her crib for both her naps. But we are terribly afraid of endangering her night sleep, which is fantastic. Can daytime naps in the crib in any way jeopardize her night sleep if she doesn't sleep during the day?

You shouldn't – mustn't – feel insecure about daytime naps in the crib. She will immediately sense your anxiety and will get the idea that something is wrong and that danger threatens. So arm yourself with an attitude of supreme confidence. Assume she will appreciate the opportunity to move up in the world! Break the happy news to her! 'Today, you get to sleep here in this great bed!' Act as though you are doing her a big favor.

Perfect a daytime jingle that doesn't contain the word night and say it when you leave (have left). Make the room as cool as you can, highlight the difference between day and night with daytime clothes, more light in the room and more noise in the house. She should feel as though she is at the center of things. She shouldn't be able to see you, but she should be able to hear you. Put on some music. Putter around in the kitchen. And as for the wolves of anxiety skulking around the bed, cast them out!

Forced to pick him up

We started the Good-Night's-Sleep Cure *three weeks ago. Our son Marcus is nine months old. At the beginning, everything went according to plan. The daytime schedule was adhered to as well and worked perfectly. (Though I have to admit that the odd night I got stuck on the jingle and had to sneak out of the room.)*

A couple of days ago, the problems started. Poop and pee leakage! Marcus woke up and was very unhappy, and I had to change him in the dark. He refused to go back to sleep in the bed. He got hysterical and I had to pick him up and comfort him. The next night it was the same story. I sat beside him, jingled and buffed for an hour and a half. I can't leave the bed when Marcus is that unhappy. The only thing that helps is sleeping beside his dad. What went wrong?

You picked him up and comforted him – and thereby saved him from his bed. Consequently, the wolf jumped up and he is still there, jaws slavering. You also ran seriously aground when you jingled in his room instead of outside the door, and when you sat (?) and buffed him for an hour and a half.

I have to give you a dressing down for not being more careful with the wonderful results you achieved. Instead, you began to question your child's sound night sleep. Marcus naturally started to do the same. He sensed mortal danger when you became insecure. And that was what drove him to despair. He was given conflicting messages and it totally confused him. You picked him up and took him away from what should have been his securely protected sleep sanctuary. That profound sense of inner security that he began to feel when he learned to trust in his parents' ability to keep the wolf at bay is gone because you have demonstrated through your actions that it is mortally dangerous for him to sleep in his own snug bed. You don't stand guard in the midst of those who are sleeping. You are in effect telling him that without your physical protection, the wolf will get him. And that of course is just not true!

Restore order! Read *Security*. Security is a way station on the road to *enjoyment* and that is not something you would want to deny your little boy, is it?

The fifteen-minute margin and the alarm clock

My daughter Scarlett is a year old. She loves waking up at 5.30 in the morning and today she didn't go back to sleep until 7.10. Can I use the fifteen minute margin and let her sleep until 7.45, even though her wake-up time is actually 7.30?

When she wakes up at 5.30, she whines more than she cries. She quiets down by herself and is silent for a few minutes, and then starts whining again. In the end, she starts to cry. Should I jingle as soon as she wakes up, or should I just let her be? I understand that I should be careful about intervening unnecessarily and that ideally she should fall back to sleep by herself.

Yes, you can fall back on the fifteen minute margin in situations like this – depending on the child's needs. It is good that she fell back to sleep on her own. This little early-morning interlude will soon be a thing of the past.

When she wakes up, it's easy for her to believe that she's slept out after a relatively long night, but she isn't. Not yet. So I think you should jingle immediately in this particular situation, even though she hasn't had time to get upset. With an information jingle x 4 – that sounds almost incidental but is nevertheless clear – tell her that it's not morning yet. Then leave her in peace. I don't think you are on the verge of falling into the over-concentration trap, but if you feel it creeping up on you, concentrate on cleaning the kitchen instead!

For children Scarlett's age (and older), an alarm clock can be a reliable aid. You can buy it together, formally appoint it the family's best friend, place it so both you and little Scarlett can hear it, and when it rings, the day begins with all the appropriate fanfare. She will learn very quickly that the day begins when the alarm goes off and not a moment before. You can then dispense with the information jingle, since it will no longer be needed.

Rock first, then buff

Is it OK to begin with your 'carriage cure' for four-month-old babies, even though my son Benjamin is seven months, and then switch to the crib and buffing? Or is it better to concentrate on buffing rather than to try with the carriage?

Greetings from a mother who is so sleep deprived she has broken out in a rash all over her face.

Yes, that will work a treat. That's how many people start off, since it is so rewarding to rock (at least I think so). But you have to work on your technique. You can read up on this in the Tool Box, where you have a complete description.

Benjamin is now so big and strong (and so mobile if you lay him down on his stomach) that he should be discreetly harnessed in the carriage if he is to spend the night there. Once his night sleep has stabilized, you can easily switch to a crib. Effective buffing (which you might not have to resort to other than to indicate that it's time to sleep) will become an extension or a recreation of rocking.

The first time you rock or buff to calm Benjamin and help him find peace, it will take its own sweet time, since he will have no idea what is going on and will ask a million questions. Don't let that scare you off. Do your homework so that you are prepared for anything. Through your actions, you will answer these questions calmly, confidently and reassuringly until Benjamin feels he has been given satisfactory answers. Then he will react with relief.

And you can then start reaping your reward. Your rash will disappear and you can begin the journey towards a good life for you all. Keep your eyes on the prize. You will regain your strength, your joie de vivre and your sleep! 'What will I do with all this free time?' you will wonder. And won't that be an easy burden to bear!

Creatures of habit

On Wednesday, in the middle of the follow-up week, I have an errand to run. I will have time to put seven-month-old Caroline down for the night, but what will happen if she wakes up? Is it OK if her dad does the jingle or will she get confused? What should we do after the follow-up week if we have to use a baby-sitter? In one month, we are going away for the weekend and will spend the night with friends. And what will happen if all three of us are away for the night? Will the jingle work if Caroline has to sleep in a strange bed?

It is quite appropriate for Dad to take a couple of nights now if he hasn't done so already. (Why hasn't he do you think?) He should work on perfecting his jingle. He will be able to do the job as well as you do and with the same effect. He should have his own jingle and be able to carry on a 'dialogue' with little Caroline that he feels really hits the mark. And it is important that you both go in and celebrate the start of a new day every morning so that you confirm each other in front of her. Both of you are standing guard against the wolf.

The lynchpin of the *Good-Night's-Sleep Cure* is the timetable. Young children are creatures of habit. They are very flexible as far as places and people are concerned, but when it comes to the timetable, their flexibility quotient is absolute zero. The fifteen minute margin is the outer limit. People are surprised over how decisively important hard and fast routines are for young children, even kids as young as two months, and this preference in children must be accorded the profound respect it deserves. Caroline will happily sleep anywhere, consent to be put to bed by anyone and accept jingles wherever she happens to be – although you should arrange for a crib or a carry cot with sides – as long as the *times* remain constant. So tattoo the schedule on your arm if you have to and make sure everyone involved knows what the drill is! Write the schedule out for them.

Perky and happy – after being put to bed

When bedtime rolls around, six-month-old Julian is often a little sleepy after his evening bottle. But when I put him down and position him, he suddenly perks up and starts to babble. Should I just leave him to it and do nothing? Most of the time, he falls asleep by himself after a few minutes. Or should I give him the confirmation jingle when he quiets down?

When he is babbling happily in the evening, don't disturb him. Sleeping every minute that he 'is supposed to' is not what's important. *What's important is that he has the prerequisites to sleep.* So give them to him, but be sure to include the bedtime laugh and all the attendant rituals. Then put him down, position him, and jingle on your way out of the room as well as from outside the door. If he falls asleep after a happy end to the day, he won't need the confirmation. And he will wake up a happy boy too!

(Continued) We put him down at eight in the evening and he wakes up around eleven. He sometimes wakes up before then, and I jump out of bed, but he quiets down before I even have time to get to the door. I am overjoyed! When he wakes up for real, I go into his room and then he cries. He is not in despair though. It's just regular crying. I give him the jingle, but then he starts to yell at the top of his lungs. Perhaps I should try to drown his voice with my own? (I can't help thinking about my poor husband, who has to get up for work at six in the morning.) I end up buffing instead and that usually quiets him down.

I bet he does yell at the top of his lungs when you suddenly roar in and start jingling in his room. Your son wonders what on earth you are doing there. And so do I!

Give him the jingle from outside the door and as you are moving away. You might disturb your husband, but he will just have to live with that during the cure. In any case, guys, like young children, are usually pretty good at turning a deaf ear to things that they don't have direct responsibility for.

Only go in if there's a crisis. And I mean a *crisis*. Then firmly reposition, hold your child in place for a few seconds with the fan and then, with a final nudge, jingle yourself out and away. Only do this once per wakeful incident! Never deliver more than one jingle on top of the one you exited with and don't stand too close to the door. Wait and listen. *Don't* just charge in. You have got to have greater confidence in your child – and, if I may say so – show him more respect.

(Continued) I wrote to you a few days ago because, even though I had administered the cure, my son still woke up frequently. You wrote back and made me understand that going in to him was absolutely forbidden and that I should jingle outside the door. That night he slept like never before. I am really thrilled over how successful we've been.

Now I am into my seventh night, and he's never been worse. He woke up constantly and at around three, he began to wail like a banshee. He screamed for over an hour (I've never heard him scream like that). I was on the verge of tears and so desperate that I gave him the pacifier. I know that was a cardinal sin and I feel sick just thinking about it. I can't get it out of my mind and I feel like a complete failure as a mother. I'm afraid I've wrecked everything – he's been waking up a lot over the last seven days and nights, but he wasn't waking up twice an hour like he was before we started the cure. What should I do?

Keep it together! For one thing, the cure is nowhere near finished yet. You are in the middle of the follow-up week and the work must continue calmly and gently. (See the chapter entitled *Security*.) For another, your son has had a little relapse, no more, and that is so common that it pretty much goes with the territory. It seems as though young children must take one last dive into the dark waters of what once was to be able to leave all that behind them for good. What confused you was that you didn't know what you should do – but actually, you do! Read up again and take heart! It's simply a matter of soldiering on, and cultivating an attitude of supreme confidence and perhaps a little more objectivity (yes, you can do it!). And remember what all this is in aid of: little Julian will be able to sleep well. And that's a gift that lasts a lifetime.

If, against expectations, this wailing continues in spite of your not having stormed into his room, you always have fanning to fall back on in emergencies. Study the Tool Box!

Don't think of yourself as a bad mother. That is not going to do anyone any good, least of all Julian. Away with the pacifier! Throw it in the garbage and forget about it. Believe in yourself. You are the best friend your child has in this world and that's how you should see yourself!

And remember: *Once is a coincidence; twice is a habit; three times is a lifestyle.*

On the run

Last night something happened that I had been dreading. My daughter Isabel, 17 months, climbed out of her crib and trotted out of her room! Since she had been screaming long and loud, I felt that I had to take her into my bed, but she wriggled around for two hours before she finally fell asleep.

Now I don't know what to do. I am in a panic about this evening, since I don't know where I should put her to bed. She has now figured out that all she has to do is climb out of the crib...

As you see, taking her into your bed is not a good idea. She won't sleep any the better for it. She wasn't trying to run away, nor was it a longing for the parental bed that made her decide to scale the wall. All she wanted to do was *climb*. So nip panic in the bud, put her to bed as you always do and administer a special mini-cure.

Reposition her in whatever way works best and hold her little body there with both hands for approximately ten seconds without saying anything (the fan). Make sure the room is dark. Conclude with a little extra pressure, get up and leave immediately without turning around or lingering at the threshold. As you move out of the room and away, deliver the goodnight jingle, which should be melodic, rhythmic, firm, confident, final and sufficiently long. Deliver four verses, one after the other with no pause in between. Then sit in the doorway and occupy yourself with something that does *not* concern her.

As soon as you hear that she is trying to clamber out of the bed, go in very quickly, put her back down again without a word and repeat the procedure described above. Keep it up as long as she does. If she calls to you and asks for things, you answer with the same jingle that you used before – the *non-sequitur* variety. Sooner or later, she will give in and go to sleep.

If she comes trotting into your room to show you that she is clever enough to climb out of bed, just take her back (she should walk herself) and repeat the procedure. Get a chair and let her climb back into bed. This will take a little time and effort. Apply a little pressure to her body and then leave with a kind but firm jingle x 4.

As already mentioned, this is a common hobby, but it will pass in a few nights – especially if you give your little human monkey access to a jungle gym during the day!

Old man

Is it possible to use the Good-Night's-Sleep Cure *on older children too, or should it be adapted somehow? Albert is 14 months old.*

My son usually falls asleep after a bottle of formula. Putting him to bed under other circumstances goes tolerably well too. But things went a lot better before. The problems occur in the wee small hours, when he wakes bright eyed and bushy tailed and we can't get him to go back to sleep. As soon as he wakes up, he stands up against the end of the bed and whimpers. The whimpering soon escalates to crying and screaming. If I go in, sit down beside him and caress him over the back, he calms down fairly quickly, but as soon as I take my hand away, he gets up again as wide awake as he can be! It doesn't matter if I stay 5, 35 or 55 minutes. He just won't go back to sleep. We often just give up (we don't have the strength to sit at his bedside for two hours every night) and take him into our bed.

Of course you can administer the *Good-Night's-Sleep Cure* to an old man! It is just the buffing that might confuse him, since his is now so big and has probably never been exposed to something like that before. He would wonder if you had all your marbles... Therefore, the order of the day is corrective positioning (see the Tool Box) and the firm, well-rehearsed jingle of the operatic 'intestinal fortitude' variety. Read up, read again, learn and prepare!

Sitting with him is not a good idea, as you have already seen. He will believe that the wolf will come for him as soon as you leave. He can't go to sleep by himself and he doesn't dare. In spite of everything, his sleep is his and his alone. You can't sleep for him. He needs help – and your confidence in him – to fall asleep initially and to go back to sleep by himself and *secure in himself.*

(To conclude) I can't express how grateful I am to you for coming up with such a superb method! When we began the cure just under a month ago, we were awake every night. The Good-Night's-Sleep Cure *gave us perfect bedtimes in only a few days. Nowadays, he still wakes up at night sometimes, but he just lies peacefully in his bed and talks to himself. There is no comparison with those nights when he would stand up in bed and scream so the windows shattered as soon as he awoke. He has even slept away from home a couple of nights, and it has gone very well too. Friends and relatives are stunned when I say, 'I'll just go put him to bed,' and come back one minute later... To sum up, we are nearly at the point where he will be sleeping twelve hours at a stretch, but it feels as though the whole family has been given a new lease on life. We now have the knowledge to carry us over the finish line!*

Wakes the whole house

We want to cure our little Beatrice, six months, but are afraid she will wake the whole house. She has a big brother, Malcolm, who has just turned two. He sleeps just fine. We were thinking that they could sleep in the same room, but that won't work, will it?

During the cure, she should of course be on her own, preferably in her own room or at least screened off from floor to ceiling, shielded from the presence of other people. However, as early as the follow-up week, when she begins to sleep through the night, she can share a room with big brother, provided that you can keep out the light effectively.

The protective instinct in young children is very strong. Malcolm will certainly wake up the first time his little sister 'demands' a jingle – but only to make sure that other people – i.e. you, the attentive parents and survival guarantors – are taking care of business so that he doesn't have to do it. Once he has assured himself that his little sister is in good hands and is receiving solid answers to her anxious questions, he will fall back into a peaceful sleep. Then heaven itself can crash to earth without waking him!

*

To Anna from Maria

I feel so frustrated. I just have to tell you what's happened today. I spoke with some parents who all had kids between two and three years of age. They complained that they didn't even have time to watch TV anymore. I couldn't understand why they didn't have time for that once the kids had gone to bed. But it turns out that these kids don't go to bed until 10.00 or 10.30! They are up at 7.00 in the morning and then they only get an hour's sleep during the day. I nearly fainted. One child, who was up until 10.30, suffered from 'night terror' and was being medicated! According to the doctor, 'night terror' could last up to the age of six.

I was so sad and angry that I didn't know where to turn. Just to calm me down, when they saw I was on the verge of literally falling over, the parents told me that their kids were really cheerful and alert. They just didn't need any more sleep! But in the next breath, they would complain that their kids couldn't sit still for more than a couple of seconds and had wild temper tantrums. One child was being tested for ADHD! The pediatrician at the children's clinic had said that this child might have sustained mild brain damage. I couldn't believe my ears! Good Lord, what is happening to children in this society?!

People like us, who have so much to thank you and the Good-Night's-Sleep Cure for, must have grown into a pretty large gang by now. For the sake of children everywhere, I hope with all my heart that there will be many, many more of us one day.

EPILOGUE FROM GASTSJÖN

Not that long ago, I would take two children into my home every other week. They ranged in age from five to eleven months. As a rule, I taught older children to sleep in their own homes, since children over a year are strongly influenced by their 'flock' and losing both parents *and* home at the same time confuses them – food for thought in a country like Sweden, where children are routinely placed in day-care far too early.

(To avoid misunderstandings: as a somewhat worn out older lady, I no longer have either the strength or the time to cure children personally.)

On the eve of the first night, I make enquiries about the child's life so far. This provides the basis for the schedule that I make up during the night. I then take care of the first night by myself and the mother sleeps in the guest house.

The children and the parents who come to me have become trapped in a vicious cycle where everyone has equally negative expectations both of themselves and of each other, and these expectations are fulfilled every night. This cycle has to be broken.

My well tested *Good-Night's-Sleep Cure* is not a variation of the grapefruit diet. ('I ate a grapefruit and weighed myself, but I hadn't lost an ounce.') It is a philosophy of life. The people who come to me have to arm themselves with complete confidence in me, their children and themselves. The *Good-Night's-Sleep Cure* doesn't just help children to sleep a little less wretchedly, which is all the parents dare to hope for. It changes lives.

Without exception, the children who come to me are chronically overtired. They are pale and whimpering, and nearly always have dark circles under their eyes. They put on a brave face, but are capable of being happy only for short periods. Their interest in food, whether it's formula or purees, is lukewarm. They get through life by half-heartedly nuzzling at the breast at all hours. Some of them are in the habit of waking up five to six times during a nine-hour night; others wake up over 25 times. The record was held by a little eight-month-old, who woke up in a screaming panic no less than 36 times! (The panic manifested itself after a two-week stint with the Controlled Crying Method.) She would nurse at her mother's breast three times an hour all night long.

All the children I have worked with in my home have one thing in common: they have never slept more than two or at the most three hours at a stretch. Consequently, neither have the mothers. But the mothers hopefully had a reserve to draw on that they had built up before their children were born. Children who have never gotten enough sleep never get the chance to build up a reserve, and what little resilience they do have is gradually broken down. After eight or nine months if not before, the parents, who up to this point have been primarily concerned with their own sleep deprivation and their generally chaotic lives, finally realize that this isn't good for the *child*.

They all turn to their local children's clinic for help, and they find that the advice they get is confusing as well as confused. They are vaguely told that all children are different. Some children need less sleep than others. Young children take the sleep they need. Some children are unusually social. That's just the way infants are. Babies belong at their mother's breasts... All these parents get pamphlets on the Controlled Crying Method. Then they try it, but most stop because they can't bear their children's hysterical screaming. Some soldier on, but soon see that what little sleep their children were once getting is being destroyed too. Some have been referred to infant psychologists, who are unable to help. (It has to be remembered that parents who really do get the help they need don't end up at my door.) Others have been given 'tranquilizing drops' – neuroleptics – which are about as tranquilizing as a general anesthetic. At this point, parents finally rebel. They do not want to drug their infant children.

'My' mothers tell me how they would want their nights to look, and even if they don't believe their dreams will come true, they have to motivate themselves. What times suit the rest of the family? What about their babies? Are they morning kids or evening kids? Once we have set the timetable, it can't be changed for the foreseeable future. It's the only way to create order out of chaos. Young children have to know what the drill is. And I assure them that *most things that have to do with children are much simpler than everyone thinks as long as there is a clearly defined goal.*

We work out how many hours of sleep their children are getting out of every 24, and some grim facts emerge. A seven-month-old baby, who needs 15 hours of sleep out of 24, has had to make do with 10. An eleven-month-old has perhaps managed 8 to 9 hours of sleep when he should have been getting 14. Most adults need approximately eight hours' sleep per night. If we superimposed 'my' infants' sleep patterns on an adult, that would mean 5 hours sleep per night, a 3-hour shortfall in other words – for an undetermined period of time. Moreover, these five hours of sleep would not be continuous, but would be interrupted two, three, four or more times by raiding the fridge, watching TV, snuggling up to one's nearest and dearest... How many adults would survive that and for how long?!

The evening ritual begins an hour before bedtime. The children bathe, eat, *laugh* – preferably until they're fit to burst. The bedtime laugh is as important for a child's well-being as formula or breast milk. Little children of four to five months are then put down on their stomach in a carriage with a tucked in sheet that has been folded in three instead of a pillow. Children this young should have breathing alarms, which the parents can buy or rent before they come. Older children can be put to bed in a crib, also with sheets folded in three to serve as pillows.

The mother, with the child on her arm, can familiarize herself with the room for a while, turn out the light, open the window a crack and pull down the blinds. If there is a pacifier in the picture, it is taken away. The child forgets all about it on the first night.

The mother then leaves and I correctively position the child – she (let's say) is on her stomach, arms up, legs stretched out, and head to the side. She is covered by a thin quilt or blanket. Then I place one hand on her back and 'buff' her little bottom with the other hand clenched in a loose fist. I work from the bottom up the length of her little body so that she gets a substantial nudge every time. On every fourth buff I apply gentle but firm pressure on her back and, if necessary, hold one finger on her neck/head simultaneously. This first *message* that I convey through my actions takes between 20 and 45 minutes to get through to a little baby who has no idea what's going on. I don't say anything. This is about the child and the child's sleep. It's not about me, and it's not about comforting the child. Actually, it's not about emotions at all.

The buffing soon relaxes the little body completely, which is of course a prerequisite for anyone to go to sleep.

The crying dies away and stops only to start up again immediately. New questions (or repeated ones) follow in the form of crying. I don't buff the whole time, and my technique varies. The lustier the crying, the firmer, the more energetic and the faster the buffing will be. If the crying is weak, the buffing will be softer and slower. As soon as the child is still and quiet, but *before* she falls asleep, I round off with gentle pressure over her back as a finale. I get up and deliver a rhythmic goodnight jingle in a friendly matter-of-fact tone of voice as I leave the room. The jingle is given as a unit with four parts, possibly six, that come one after the other. The first part comes when I leave the bed and go out the door. The rest are delivered from just outside the door and as I move away.

The goodnight jingle, which is always (and only) given at night and which never varies, will soon trigger a conditioned reflex in the child. She will fall asleep flat on her stomach. Naturally, we don't come that far on the first night, but more often than not that goal is reached as early as the second or the third. (In my experience, infants sleep their absolute best in the prone position, and once they discover the joy of sleeping on their stomachs, they seldom change.)

Many parents have adopted my own jingle, which is simplicity itself:

'Nightie-NIGHT-Sleep-So-TIGHT.' It can sound light and happy, reassuring and calm, caressing and sweet, firm and slightly irritated, bright or dark, loud or soft, melodic or nagging and monotonous. It all depends on the kind of 'conversation' we're having. The answers are tailored to the child's questions. This is how a dialogue is conducted with the child.

After the jingle, which, at the beginning, results in renewed crying, I listen to the child carefully. Is the crying gradually dying away? If so, I interpret it as a *reaction* to the message I have conveyed. There is no law against reacting – nor should there be, since young children's reactions should be respected not silenced. If, however, the crying is cranking up and new, anxious, over-excited questions are being posed, I give new answers – in the form of reassuring reminders.

In the former case, I wait a little longer and then give a so-called confirmation jingle when the child is silent but not yet asleep. This jingle is soft and delicate, and tells the child that all is right with the world. She can lie where she is and sleep the sleep of the just. She need not give the wolf so much as a passing thought because the only thing that people do here is fall peacefully asleep. The confirmation is literally the last word and it follows the child into dream land *as a confirmation.*

In the latter case, once the first message is conveyed, I give as many reassuring reminders as are necessary to convince the child that I am fully capable of keeping the wolf at bay. I reposition again, buff again, give the jingle again as many times as the child asks – and then once more until the confirmation jingle brings everything to a contented end and the child falls asleep in peace.

I 'rock' infants in carriages according to the same principle. I reposition as described above and pull the carriage rhythmically and quickly back and forth and give the carriage a good jerk in each direction so that those little bodies relax. It's a technique that takes practice, just like the jingle. Remember that any anxious, insecure hesitation that manifests itself while you are trying convey a soothing message, be it in action or in word, will immediately exacerbate the child's anxiety. Then danger *really* threatens!

The louder the crying, the worse the anxiety and the firmer and more powerful the rocking should be. If the crying is soft, only gentle, slow rocking is needed to get the child to quiet down. And a quiet, relaxed and calm child is what you are aiming for. *Young children should be calmed where they are lying* so that they dare to sleep securely. That is always the overriding goal.

I round off the rocking with a few quick shakes of the carriage handle while the child is still awake.

The big breakthrough comes when the child no longer connects falling asleep (or the occasional wakeful moment which she will take care of herself) with danger.

During the night I keep watch so that I can instantly give answers to questions as soon as the child wakes up. I repeat the message, give as many reminders as necessary and finally give the confirmation jingle until it is peacefully accepted.

During that first twelve-hour night (or whatever has been decided), children can wake up ten to twenty times and pose their anxious questions for anything from 30 seconds to an hour at a time. I answer as many times as it takes – and then once more.

The second night is when these kids set personal records for continuous sleep, even if it's only four to five hours. The number of times they wake up and the length of time they are awake usually fall by half.

The third night, these statistics are halved again, and the children sleep continuously for seven, eight or nine hours, and total night sleep begins to approach the target.

On the fourth twelve-hour night, the kids don't wake up that often, one to three times or not at all. They quiet down immediately when they hear the jingle, even if they don't go back to sleep right away – especially not in the wee small hours. But these children are starting to feel secure even then. They are beginning to believe that the wolf isn't coming for them and they can allow themselves to enjoy lying snug and warm in their beds. By this stage, buffing has been replaced by the jingle in all its various tones of voice.

From here on in, buffing should be regarded as an emergency measure.

And overusing it is not a trap you want to fall into, since it doesn't take young children long to figure out how good buffing feels. Imagine how quickly an adult might get hooked on being massaged all night. This, however, is not really what we want to achieve!

There is also a risk that the goodnight jingle from outside the door might come to be regarded as rather entertaining if Mom and Dad don't think ahead. The jingle conveys *the message, a reminder and a confirmation –* and nothing else. It is not supposed to keep the child awake.

The schedule I outline for the day is based on ensuring that a child gets enough food and enough sleep. I start off with night sleep, which, let's say, we want to run from seven at night until seven the next morning. Even after a long night, young children are tired after being awake for around two hours, so we would splice in a nap of either 45 minutes or an hour and a half. Sleep periods that coincide with natural sleep rhythms are exactly 5 minutes, 20 minutes, 45 minutes, 1.5 hours, 2 hours, 3 hours, after which it is easy to wake children, even if they don't wake up by themselves.

Children should eat at three-and-a-half-hour intervals, four at most, from start to start and from five months and up, meals should not last more than 30 minutes.

I splice in four meals plus an evening top up from the bottle and/or breast, which comes last thing before bed and can be given as little as an hour after dinner.

A nap of 1.5 hours (or whatever is appropriate depending on the child's total sleep needs) can be planned for the early afternoon. A six-month-old baby needs approximately 15 hours of sleep, a seven to eight-month-old 14.5, a nine to ten-month-old 14, and a one-year-old 13.5.

In the morning, 'my' parents announce the start of the day with much fanfare at the appointed time. A new day has come! Waking up should be great fun, just as much fun as going to sleep is going to be. The latter paves the way for the former. The schedule must be adhered to with a fifteen minute margin of error in both directions so that you can splice in 'wake-up calls' while a child is soundly asleep or at least quiet. (Not if a child is crying however. Then it's a matter of questions and answers.)

During the *Good-Night's-Sleep Cure*, these children undergo a metamorphosis. Over the first two days, their fatigue rises to the surface – fatigue that Nature's imperatives had forced them to suppress. No matter how much anxiety, stress and sleep deprivation young children are burdened with, they still have to grow, develop, learn and process new impressions with all their senses working flat out every waking moment. They can't take mental holidays. Their conditioning gives them no peace. When they finally get the rest and the mental relief they need, fatigue becomes wholesome sleepiness. They rub their eyes and yawn. Their pallor vanishes and roses start to color their cheeks.

On the third day eating problems start to subside and appetites increase. The shock to their stomachs can lead to constipation, and prune puree is the antidote, a jar a day. Fixed meal times with a clear beginning and a clear end – 'thanks for the meal!' – make life easier. Their clinginess disappears and they gather strength. Motor skills become more reliable. The children 'talk' with new, contented sounds, sometimes from their beds, and no sound is more beautiful. Way back when, human beings began the day with a song!

The journey to my door is long and hard, but the journey home on the fourth day is a thrilling adventure. Dads who have stayed home are reunited with their kids, and they usually exclaim, 'We have got a whole new little person here!' Development literally explodes. The whole family find themselves on an upward spiral that becomes just as self-perpetuating as the downward one was. And everyone concerned understands what I mean when I say, *Young children should be enjoyed – and enjoy themselves.*

The *Good-Night's-Sleep Cure* continues with a follow-up week at home, which should be as uneventful and simple as possible. All the routines stabilize and solidify. The odd sliver of anxiety remains. The hour of the wolf (between 4 and 6 in the morning) can be a tough nut to crack, and makes its presence felt. One or two daytime naps have yet to find their slots. Parents are sometimes tempted to change the schedule before it has had time to stabilize, but that is as confusing as switching the numbers around on the clock face before a child has learned to tell the time.

At this point, the kids should be sleeping in their own rooms or in screened off corners with blackout blinds from floor to ceiling, since the presence of their parents will otherwise disturb them. It doesn't matter in the least if the child *hears* them – quite the contrary in fact. Seeing them, however, makes a child decidedly anxious and/or curious of course.

Long submerged wreckage will rise to the surface. Various stubborn ailments that have lain dormant for weeks or months will bloom and vanish. A child can also have a relapse and succumb to the odd wretched bout of survival anxiety and then give it the heave-ho for ever. A child can have a breakdown at bed time in the mistaken belief that all the good times are over and will never return. But she soon realizes that more fun stuff will happen the next day, and the day after that, and the day after that... Existence becomes predictable and contented sleep ensues.

When, after a month long cure, 'my' children are 'finished' so to speak and survival anxiety has given way to *real* security – the kind of security that the children carry within themselves – they have been known to crawl or walk to their cribs, right in the middle of the evening festivities, and look beseechingly at their loving progenitors as if to say, 'Put me to bed please!'

The self-esteem and confidence of the parents increases in step with the child's.

One month after the start of the cure, the pennies have dropped all the way up the line. These children have become their own little clocks. The schedule provides security for all parties. Life is a walk in the park that can be planned and enjoyed. These kids can predict their days and they greet each one of them joyously. Crying is a thing of the past, and sleeping and eating are activities that can be pursued anywhere as long as the timetable is respected. Good night sleep is here to stay. Their independence is massive. These children are not just secure little people; they are *free* as well and everyone can see it.

These children have resources to draw on. Teething is no longer unpleasant. It just itches a little so it feels good to gnaw on some sugar-free crisp bread. They have endurance. Whatever has to be contended with is no longer unbearably stressful. Those days when these kids were so exhausted that everything was too much are gone forever, as are the days when their moms never got out of their nightgowns and would burst into tears at the thought of a family get-together or a night on the town. These children can take a new tooth or a bout of fever in their stride, not to mention the demanding balancing act that standing entails. And walking. All by themselves. Without wobbling on tired, uncertain legs. Once they're slept out, life is *always* fun!

And that's the way it should be. Young children should be courageous and happy. Joie de vivre and a lust for life dwell within them. Human beings with their relatively delicate constitutions haven't survived as a species by being weak, helpless and pathetic. They haven't come to rule the earth because they are objects of pity. They are not born to succumb to life's tribulations, but to explore, master and change their reality, their living conditions and their world. The *iron will* that young children possess and that their parents sometimes complain about is the reason the adults themselves are still walking their earth.

Naturally, my work can be sabotaged. The victims are the children. The survival anxiety that took four days to banish can be reinstated in five minutes. During the follow-up week, if the parents themselves pose questions in the hope that their *children* will provide those reassuring answers, they are in effect transferring their own intrusive fears to their children and fishing for reassurance – and their children will react by immediately sensing danger. Again. For if the parents can't guarantee their own survival, how can they guarantee their children's?

These young children would never take my *Good-Night's-Sleep Cure* to heart so eagerly as soon as they receive satisfactory answers to their anxious questions – and from a stranger to boot – if they were not desperate to avoid having to fear the wolf and wanted nothing more than to dare to sleep well.

Those parents who administer my *Good-Night's-Sleep Cure* with me or at home by themselves might not all manage to once and for all shoot the wolf, but they do manage to keep him at a safe distance. Their kids get their sleep night after night, year after year. (As far as I know, out of the about eight hundred children that I have worked with, I have only failed with two, and these kids were on neuroleptics. They should have been de-toxed first.)

Does it sound difficult? Do you think that my *Good-Night's-Sleep Cure* is complicated and demanding?

It is. It demands personal commitment. It demands your heart, your love and your concentration. It demands your indefatigable good will, which places the focus on your child's long term interests rather than your – and society's – short term ones. It is based on a certain view of children – that they are human beings of flesh and blood, rather than recreational accessories that are always subordinated to the whims of the patriarchal labor market. Young children are not stuffed animals to be played with when you have nothing better to do. They must be treated with loving respect, and this respect manifests itself through your actions.

The *Good-Night's-Sleep Cure* represents a philosophy of life that requires human empathy, constructive attention, unshakable personal responsibility, sound creative thinking and long term planning. In a nutshell, it demands *parenting that reassures.*

Gastsjön, Jämtland and Stockholm, Sweden, March 2009
Anna Wahlgren

A final word from a mother, Claudia

Claudia wrote to me after she and her husband had cured their little baby by themselves with the help of the first Swedish edition of *A Good Night's Sleep* that was published in 2005. It is with joy and gratitude that I give her the last word of this book:

We have been struck dumb by the effect your method has had on our little boy. We are so tremendously grateful that you are around and have dedicated your life to this important work.

We have gotten ourselves a fantastic little guy who eats like a horse, sleeps like a log and is so happy and secure his every waking moment. He radiates joy!

Today he is exactly 18 months old, and we started your cure a week ago. After more than 17 months of pestering, examinations and general chaos at the local children's clinic our pride and joy started to eat with the heartiest of appetites already on the second day of the cure. When we put him to bed in the evening, he falls asleep with a contented sigh and doesn't so much as peep when we leave the room.

All the advice we have been given by the clinic has turned out to be worthless and probably exposed him to even more wolves.

We are so deliriously happy. Best of all, we can really see how our little boy is developing by leaps and bounds – talking among other things – and how incredibly secure he feels in his routines and how proud he is of them.

Our son is bursting with happiness and energy. Only a week ago, our days were one long ordeal of fatigue, coaxing, whining and despair.

THANK YOU!